An
Illustrated
Review
of the
REPRODUCTIVE SYSTEM

Glenn F. Bastian

 HarperCollins*CollegePublishers*

Executive Editor: Bonnie Roesch
Cover Designer: Kay Petronio
Production Manager: Bob Cooper
Printer and Binder: Malloy Lithographing, Inc.
Cover Printer: The Lehigh Press, Inc.

AN ILLUSTRATED REVIEW OF THE REPRODUCTIVE SYSTEM

by Glenn F. Bastian

94 95 96 9 8 7 6 5 4 3 2

To
Claire and George Dix

CONTENTS

LIST OF TOPICS & ILLUSTRATIONS

Text: One page of text is devoted to each of the following topics. *Illustrations are listed in italics.*

PREFACE

An Illustrated Review of Anatomy and Physiology is a series of ten books written to help students effectively review the structure and function of the human body. Each book in the series is devoted to a different body system.

My objective in writing these books is to make very complex subjects accessible and nonthreatening by presenting material in manageable-size bits (one topic per page) with clear, simple illustrations to assist the many students who are primarily visual learners. Designed to supplement established texts, they may be used as a student aid to jog the memory, to quickly recall the essentials of each major topic, and to practice naming structures in preparation for exams.

INNOVATIVE FEATURES OF THE BOOK

(1) Each major topic is confined to one page of text.

A unique feature of this book is that each topic is confined to one page and the material is presented in outline form with the key terms in boldface or italic typeface. This makes it easy to scan quickly the major points of any given topic. The student can easily get an overview of the topic and then zero in on a particular point that needs clarification.

(2) Each page of text has an illustration on the facing page.

Because each page of text has its illustration on the facing page, there is no need to flip through the book looking for the illustration that is referred to in the text ("see Figure X on page xx"). The purpose of the illustration is to clarify a central idea discussed in the text. The images are simple and clear, the lines are bold, and the labels are in a large type. Each illustration deals with a well-defined concept, allowing for a more focused study.

PHYSIOLOGY TOPICS (1 text page : 1 illustration)
Each main topic in physiology is limited to one page of text with one supporting illustration on the facing page.

ANATOMY TOPICS (1 text page : several illustrations)

For complex anatomical structures a good illustration is more valuable than words. So, for topics dealing with anatomy, there are often several illustrations for one text topic.

(3) Unlabeled illustrations have been included.

In Part II, all illustrations have been repeated without their labels. This allows a student to test his or her visual knowledge of the basic concepts.

(4) A Pronunciation Guide has been included.

Phonetic spellings of unfamiliar terms are listed in a separate section, unlike other textbooks where they are usually found in the glossary or spread throughout the text. The student may use this guide for pronunciation drill or as a quick review of basic vocabulary.

(5) A glossary has been included.

Most textbooks have glossaries that include terms for all of the systems of the body. It is convenient to have all of the key terms for one system in a single glossary.

ACKNOWLEDGMENTS

I would like to thank the reviewers of the manuscript for this book who carefully critiqued the text and illustrations for their effectiveness: William Kleinelp, Middlesex County College; Robert Smith, University of Missouri, St. Louis, and St. Louis Community College, Forest Park; and Pamela Monaco, Molloy College. Their help and advice are greatly appreciated. Kay Petronio is to be commended for her handsome cover design and Bob Cooper has my gratitude for keeping the production moving smoothly. I would also like to thank my wife, Katherine Waynick Bastian, for her steadfast help and encouragement. Finally, I am greatly indebted to my editor, Bonnie Roesch, for her willingness to try a new idea, and for her support throughout this project. I invite students and instructors to send any comments and suggestions for enhancements or changes to this book to me, in care of HarperCollins, so that future editions can continue to meet your needs.

Glenn Bastian

Male Reproductive System

MALE REPRODUCTIVE SYSTEM / Overview

INTRODUCTION

The Aging Process The human body is a temporary structure. With age, fundamental changes occur, such as hardening and loss of elasticity of the connective tissues and the artery walls, deterioration and loss of neurons, and a decrease in the functioning of the immune system. Although medical science has learned to cure infectious diseases and control many metabolic disorders, the maximum age which may be reached is a little over 100.

Continuity of the Species If a species is to continue, while individuals die, there must be a mechanism for the formation of new individuals. There are two basic methods for producing off-spring: asexual reproduction and sexual reproduction.

Asexual Reproduction Asexual reproduction is any method of forming new offspring that does not involve the union of two gametes (sperm and ovum). It is used by microorganisms, many plants, and lower animals. For example, bacteria split into two roughly equal halves by a process called *fission*, yeast cells proliferate by a process called *budding*, and fungi form *spores*.

Sexual Reproduction Sexual reproduction involves two fundamental processes: gametogenesis (the production of gametes) and fertilization (the fusion of gametes). The gametes formed have half the normal chromosome number, so when they fuse during fertilization the normal chromosome number is restored. All gametes formed are genetically different from their parent cell and from each other, so all new organisms are genetically unique.

MALE REPRODUCTIVE SYSTEM

Testes The testes (singular: testis) produce *spermatozoa* (sperm) and the hormone *testosterone*.
Seminiferous Tubules Each testis is divided into about 250 compartments called *lobules*, and each lobule contains one to three highly coiled tubules called *seminiferous tubules*. Spermatozoa are formed in the walls of these tubules by a process called *spermatogenesis*.

Spermatogenesis

Spermatogonia are diploid cells formed in the testes during embryonic development. At puberty, under the influence of FSH (secreted by the anterior pituitary gland), they become active and differentiate into *primary spermatocytes*. Each primary spermatocyte undergoes two meiotic divisions, forming four *spermatids* (immature sperm). Spermatids undergoes *spermiogenesis*, resulting in the formation of *spermatozoa* (mature sperm).

Accessory Structures

Ducts Spermatozoa migrate from the seminiferous tubules to a highly coiled tube called the *ductus epididymis* located just outside each testis; here they are stored and become fully motile. During ejaculation, the spermatozoa from each testis travel via the *ductus deferens* and *ejaculatory duct* to the *urethra*. They exit the body via the urethra, which passes through the penis.
Glands Several glands secrete fluids into the ducts, forming *semen* (fluid plus sperm). These glands are the two *seminal vesicles*, the *prostate gland*, and the two *bulbourethral glands*.
Penis The penis is the male organ of copulation. It contains three cylindrical masses of spongy tissue that can become engorged with blood, causing erection.

Hormonal Control

Five hormones control male reproductive functions: *GnRH* (gonadotropin-releasing hormone), *FSH* (follicle-stimulating hormone), *LH* (luteinizing hormone), *inhibin*, and *testosterone*.

FERTILIZATION

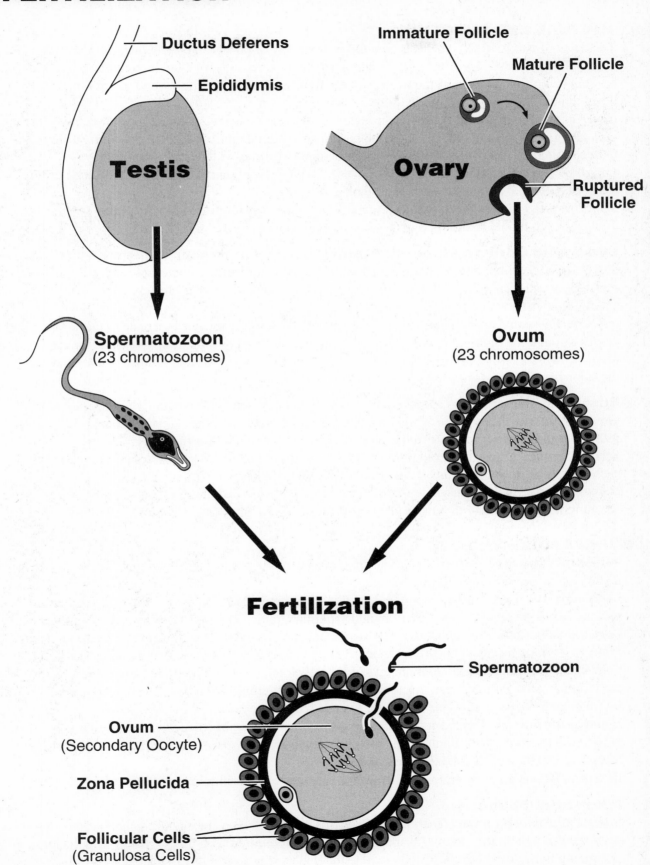

MALE REPRODUCTIVE SYSTEM / Testes

STRUCTURE AND FUNCTION

Testes (Testicles)   The testes are the primary sex organs of the male; they are also called the *male gonads*. These paired oval glands are about two inches long and one inch in diameter, and have the same embryonic origin as the ovaries of the female. During the the seventh month of fetal development, they descend into the scrotum through the inguinal canals.

Coverings   Two tissue layers cover the testes: the tunica vaginalis and the tunica albuginea. The *tunica vaginalis* is an outpocketing of the peritoneum, formed during the descent of the testes. The *tunica albuginea* is a dense white fibrous tissue that is internal to the tunica vaginalis.

Lobules   The tunica albuginea extends inward, forming septa (partitions) that divide each testis into about 250 internal compartments called lobules.

Seminiferous Tubules   Each lobule contains one to three tightly coiled tubules called seminiferous tubules. Each tubule is about 28 inches long when uncoiled.

Spermatic Cord and Inguinal Canal   Sperm is transported from the testes into the abdominal cavity within a tubule called the *ductus deferens*. The ductus deferens with its associated structures (testicular artery, autonomic nerves, veins, lymphatic vessels, and cremaster muscle) is called the spermatic cord. The *cremaster muscle* consists of skeletal muscle fibers; it elevates the testes during sexual arousal and on exposure to cold. The spermatic cord ascends in the scrotum and passes through the *inguinal canal*. The canal is about two inches long; it originates at the *deep inguinal ring* (a slitlike opening in the aponeurosis of the transversus abdominis muscle) and ends at the *superficial inguinal ring* (a triangular opening in the aponeurosis of the external oblique muscle).

Scrotum   The scrotum is a skin-covered pouch that contains the testes and their accessory structures. Because the scrotum is outside the abdominal cavity, it provides an environment that is about 3°C lower than the normal core body temperature; this is essential for the survival of sperm.

Scrotal Septum   The scrotal septum is a vertical partition that divides the scrotum into two sacs, each containing a single testis. It consists of superficial fascia and dartos muscle.

Dartos Muscle   Dartos muscle is found in the scrotal septum and in the subcutaneous tissue of the scrotum; it contains smooth muscle fibers and causes wrinkling of the scrotum.

SEMINIFEROUS TUBULES

Walls of Tubules   The walls of the seminiferous tubules consist of two types of cells: spermatogenic (sperm-producing) cells and sustentacular cells.

Spermatogenic Cells   The spermatogenic cells lining the walls of the seminiferous tubules are in various stages of development. They include spermatogonia, spermatocytes, and spermatids.

Sustentacular Cells (Sertoli Cells)   The sustentacular cells extend from the outer basement membrane to the lumen (inner fluid-filled space). They have many functions relating to sperm production, such as the support and nourishment of the developing cells. Immature sperm are embedded in the luminal membranes of sustentacular cells before being released into the lumen. When stimulated by follicle-stimulating hormone (FSH) these cells secrete the hormone inhibin.

Blood–testis Barrier   Tight junctions between the outer regions of adjacent sustentacular cells form a blood–testis barrier. This is important because the developing sperm have surface antigens that are recognized as foreign by the immune system.

Basement Membrane   A basement membrane surrounds each seminiferous tubule.

Interstitial Space

Interstitial Endocrinocytes (Interstitial Cells of Leydig)   Clusters of interstitial endocrinocytes are scattered throughout the interstitial space between the seminiferous tubules. When stimulated by luteinizing hormone (LH), these cells secrete the male sex hormone testosterone.

TESTES
Anatomy

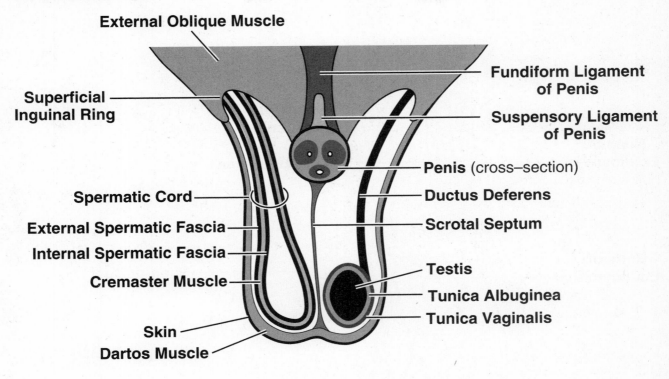

External Oblique Muscle

Superficial Inguinal Ring

Spermatic Cord

External Spermatic Fascia

Internal Spermatic Fascia

Cremaster Muscle

Skin

Dartos Muscle

Fundiform Ligament of Penis

Suspensory Ligament of Penis

Penis (cross–section)

Ductus Deferens

Scrotal Septum

Testis

Tunica Albuginea

Tunica Vaginalis

Location

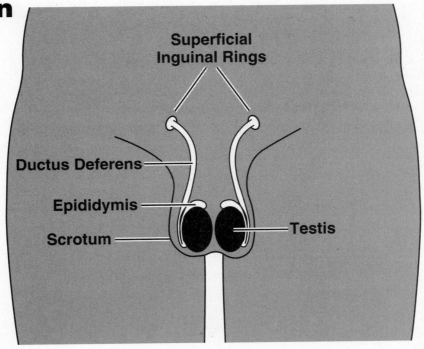

Superficial Inguinal Rings

Ductus Deferens

Epididymis

Scrotum

Testis

TESTES : Tubules
Sagittal section of a testis

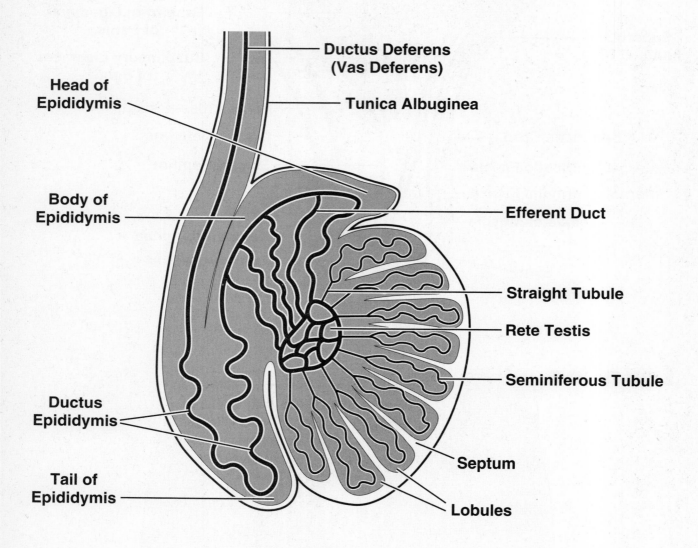

Ductus Deferens
(Vas Deferens)

Head of
Epididymis

Tunica Albuginea

Body of
Epididymis

Efferent Duct

Straight Tubule

Rete Testis

Seminiferous Tubule

Ductus
Epididymis

Tail of
Epididymis

Septum

Lobules

SEMINIFEROUS TUBULES

An Area Of Testis (cross–section)

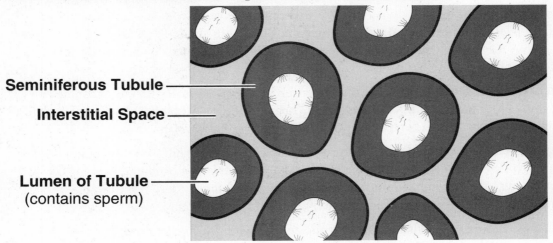

Seminiferous Tubule

Interstitial Space

Lumen of Tubule
(contains sperm)

Wall of Tubule (detail)

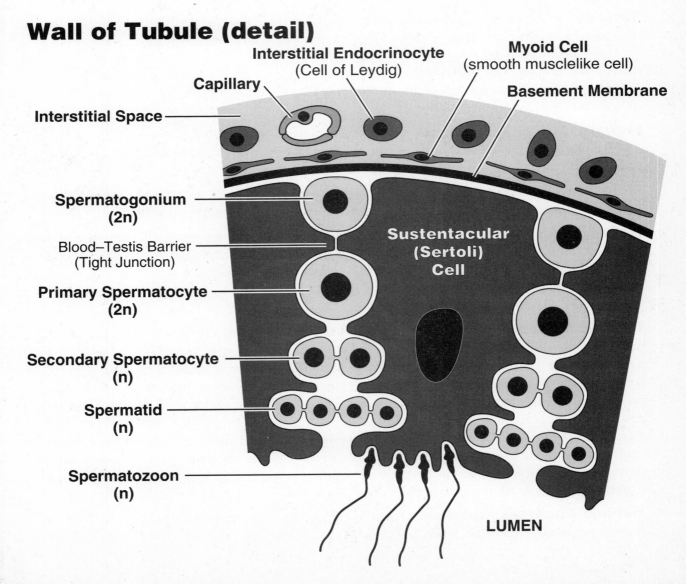

Interstitial Endocrinocyte
(Cell of Leydig)

Capillary

Myoid Cell
(smooth musclelike cell)

Basement Membrane

Interstitial Space

Spermatogonium
(2n)

Blood–Testis Barrier
(Tight Junction)

Primary Spermatocyte
(2n)

Sustentacular
(Sertoli)
Cell

Secondary Spermatocyte
(n)

Spermatid
(n)

Spermatozoon
(n)

LUMEN

MALE REPRODUCTIVE SYSTEM / Gametogenesis

CHROMOSOMES

In a nondividing cell, DNA and associated proteins are loosely packed and form a network of material called *chromatin*. During cell division, DNA and certain proteins condense and coil into rod-shaped bodies called *chromosomes*. Each chromosome contains a single DNA molecule. A gene is a portion of a DNA molecule. There are 23 different types of chromosomes in each body cell (23 pairs) and a total of about 100,000 genes.

Chromosome Number   The diploid number (abbreviated $2n$) is 46 (23 chromosome pairs); the haploid number (abbreviated n) is 23 (unpaired chromosomes). All body cells have the diploid number of chromosomes; gametes (sperm or ova) have the haploid number.

Homologous Chromosomes   One member of each pair of chromosomes is inherited from each parent; each chromosome pair has a maternal and a paternal chromosome. They are said to be homologous because they contain similar genes arranged in the same order. For example, if one chromosome contained a gene for eye color, the other would also contain a gene for eye color.

Chromatids   Before cell division, DNA duplicates, forming identical chromatids. During prophase of mitosis and meiosis I, each chromatid pair is held together by a small spherical body called a *centromere*.

Tetrads   During meiosis I, homologous chromosomes (each consisting of two identical chromatids) line up on either side of the equatorial plane; each four-chromatid grouping is called a *tetrad*.

STAGES OF GAMETOGENESIS

Gametogenesis is the production of gametes (sperm or ova). It consists of three cell divisions: mitosis, meiosis I, and meiosis II.

Mitosis   The first stage of gametogenesis is the mitosis (proliferation) of *primordial germ cells*. These diploid cells are called *spermatogonia* in males and *oogonia* in females. Some of the daughter cells differentiate into *primary spermatocytes* or *primary oocytes*.

Meiosis I   Primary spermatocytes or primary oocytes undergo meiosis I, forming *secondary spermatocytes* or *secondary oocytes*, which have the haploid chromosome number (23).

Meiosis II   Secondary spermatocytes or secondary oocytes undergo meiosis II, forming *spermatids* or an *ovum*. The spermatids differentiate into *spermatozoa*. Completion of meiosis II occurs after fertilization in females; the resulting cell is called a mature ovum.

RESULTS OF GAMETOGENESIS

Genetic Variability   During meiosis I, two events contribute to the genetic variability of the daughter cells: crossing-over and random distribution.

Crossing–over   During meiosis I, homologous chromosomes become arranged in homologous pairs, forming tetrads. At this time, corresponding segments of homologous chromosomes may overlap, break, and exchange genes. The result is a new chromatid, containing segments of both maternal and paternal genetic material.

Random Distribution of Homologous Chromosomes   After crossing-over occurs, homologous chromosomes move to opposite poles and the cell divides. Some maternal and some paternal chromosomes end up in each cell. Over eight million different combinations of maternal and paternal chromosomes can result from the random distribution of these chromosomes during meiosis I.

Haploid Gametes   The gametes formed as the result of gametogenesis have the haploid number of chromosomes. So, when two gametes fuse during fertilization, a diploid cell results.

GAMETOGENESIS

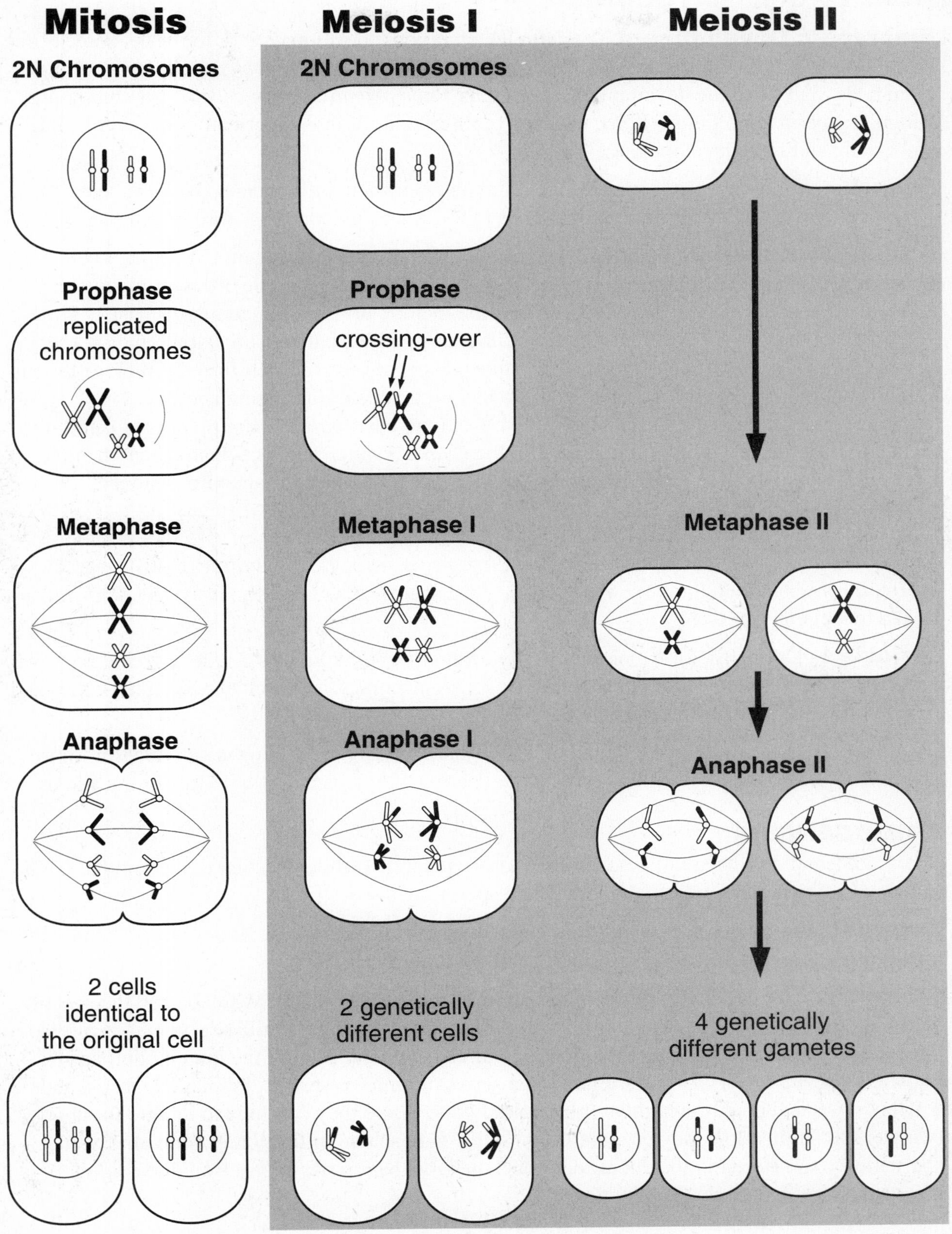

Mitosis

2N Chromosomes

Prophase
replicated chromosomes

Metaphase

Anaphase

2 cells identical to the original cell

Meiosis I

2N Chromosomes

Prophase
crossing-over

Metaphase I

Anaphase I

2 genetically different cells

Meiosis II

Metaphase II

Anaphase II

4 genetically different gametes

MALE REPRODUCTIVE SYSTEM / Spermatogenesis

MITOSIS OF SPERMATOGONIA

Embryonic Development Early in the embryonic development of the male, some of the endoderm cells lining the yolk sac differentiate into *primordial germ cells*. These primordial germ cells migrate to the developing testes and become *primitive germ cells* or *spermatogonia* (singular: spermatogonium). Some mitosis (proliferation) of these spermatogonia occurs during embryonic and fetal development.

Puberty Following birth, spermatogonia remain dormant until puberty (between ages 10 and 17). At puberty, mitosis of spermatogonia resumes; it usually continues throughout life.

A Clone Of Spermatogonia From each original spermatogonium, a clone of cells (a population of identical cells) is produced. Most of the cells in the clone differentiate into *primary spermatocytes*, which later undergo the first meiotic division of spermatogenesis. However, if all of the cells in the clone were to follow this pathway, there soon would be no spermatagonia to continue the process. For this reason, at least one cell from each clone reverts to being an undifferentiated spermatogonium that is capable of producing another clone.

In the testes, primary spermatocytes move from the outer *basal compartments* of seminiferous tubules, through the tight junctions, into the *central compartments*, which extend from the tight junctions to the lumen of the tubule. Meiosis occurs in the central compartments.

MEIOSIS OF SPERMATOCYTES

During two successive cell divisions, each primary spermatocyte divides into two *secondary spermatocytes* and then into four *spermatids*. As a spermatocyte divides, its descendents remain linked by *cytoplasmic bridges*.

Meiosis I During the first meiotic division, primary spermatocytes divide, forming secondary spermatocytes (haploid cells). Each cell has 23 chromosomes, and each chromosome consists of two chromatids joined by a centromere.

Meiosis II During the second meiotic division, secondary spermatocytes divide, forming spermatids (haploid cells). At this time, linked chromatids separate, becoming chromosomes.

SPERMIOGENESIS

Spermatids mature (differentiate) into spermatozoa (sperm) while attached to the luminal membranes of sustentacular cells, a process called spermiogenesis.

Spermatids Each spermatid develops into a single spermatozoon. It develops a head with an acrosome (enzyme-containing granule) and a flagellum (tail).

Spermatozoa A single spermatogonium produces about 500 spermatozoa and the process takes about 10 weeks. A young adult may produce several hundred million spermatozoa per day. Spermatozoa are released from the sustentacular cells into the fluid of the lumen (a process known as *spermiation*). They pass through a series of tubules (straight tubule, rete testis, and efferent duct) and enter the highly coiled epididymis, where they continue to mature for about two weeks. At this time they become fully motile and capable of fertilizing an ovum. Some spermatozoa are stored in the ductus deferens, the tube that carries sperm from the epididymis to the ejaculatory duct during ejaculation.

SPERMATOGENESIS

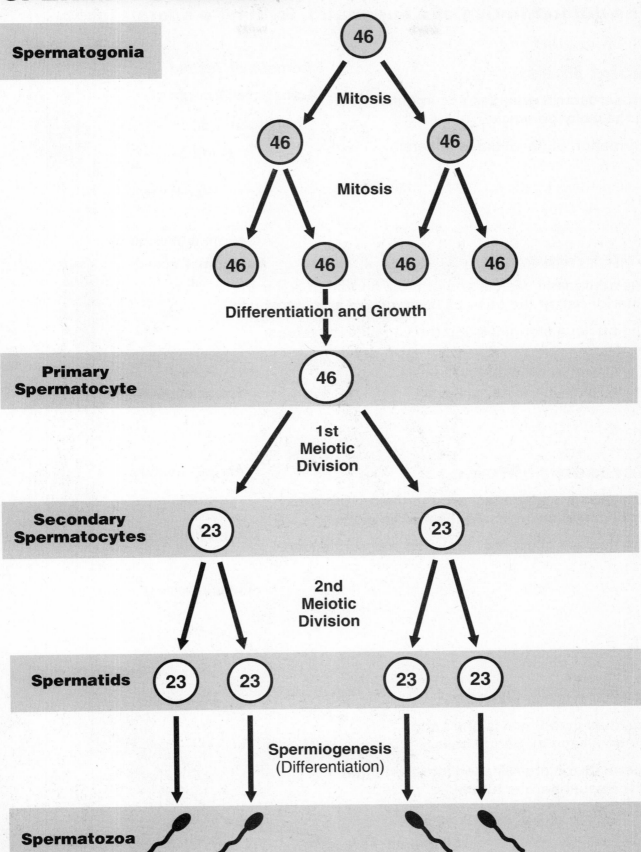

Spermatogonia

46

Mitosis

46   46

Mitosis

46   46   46   46

Differentiation and Growth

Primary Spermatocyte   46

1st Meiotic Division

Secondary Spermatocytes   23   23

2nd Meiotic Division

Spermatids   23   23   23   23

Spermiogenesis (Differentiation)

Spermatozoa

SPERMIOGENESIS
The differentiation of a spermatid, forming a spermatozoon.

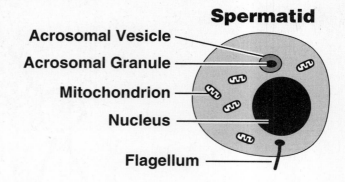

Spermatid

Acrosomal Vesicle
Acrosomal Granule
Mitochondrion
Nucleus
Flagellum

Golgi Phase

Proacrosomal granules accumulate in the Golgi complex.

Formation of flagellum is initiated.

Cap Phase

The acrosomal vesicle and granule spread to cover the anterior half of the nucleus, forming the acrosomal cap.

The nucleus elongates and the flagellum develops.

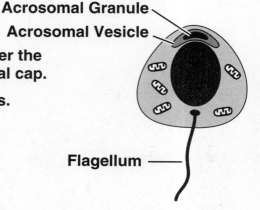

Acrosomal Granule
Acrosomal Vesicle

Flagellum

Acrosomal Phase

Mitochondria aggregate around the proximal end of the flagellum, forming the middle piece.

The nucleus becomes elongated and condensed.

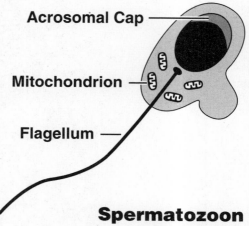

Acrosomal Cap

Mitochondrion

Flagellum

Maturation Phase

Residual cytoplasm is shed and phagocytized by Sertoli cells.

Spermatozoa are released into the lumen of the seminiferous tubule.

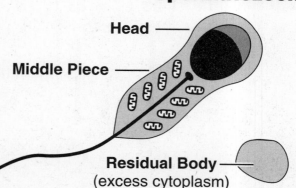

Spermatozoon

Head

Middle Piece

Flagellum

Residual Body
(excess cytoplasm)

HUMAN SPERMATOZOON

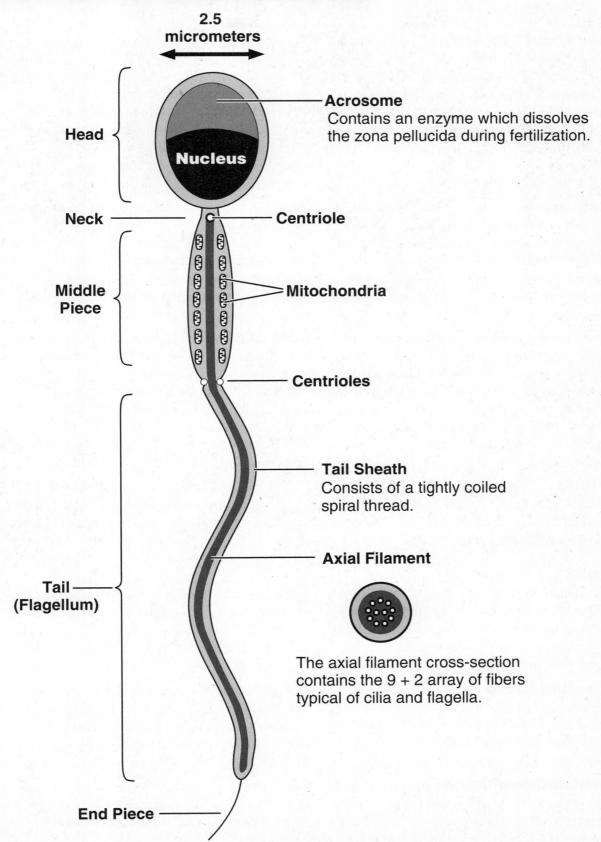

2.5 micrometers

Head

Nucleus

Acrosome
Contains an enzyme which dissolves the zona pellucida during fertilization.

Neck — **Centriole**

Middle Piece

Mitochondria

Centrioles

Tail (Flagellum)

Tail Sheath
Consists of a tightly coiled spiral thread.

Axial Filament

The axial filament cross-section contains the 9 + 2 array of fibers typical of cilia and flagella.

End Piece

MALE REPRODUCTIVE SYSTEM / Ducts and Glands

DUCTS

Ducts and Tubules of the Testes

Seminiferous Tubule A seminiferous tubule is a tightly coiled tube about 28 inches long when uncoiled; the two testes contain about 250 yards of these tubules. Each lobule in a testis contains one to three seminiferous tubules. It is the site of spermatogenesis (sperm production).

Straight Tubule A straight tubule is a tube leading from a seminiferous tubule to the rete testis.

Rete Testis The rete testis is a network of tubes in each testis (*rete* = net or meshwork). It receives spermatozoa from the straight tubules.

Efferent Ducts The efferent ducts are a series of coiled tubes that transport spermatozoa from the rete testis to the epididymis.

Epididymis (*epi* = above; *didymos* = testis) The epididymis is a comma-shaped structure about 1.5 inches long that is loosely attached to the outside of each testis.

Ductus Epididymis (plural: epididymides) The epididymis of each testis contains a highly coiled tube called the ductus epididymis, which is about 6 yards long when uncoiled. It consists of the head (superior portion), the body (midportion), and the tail (inferior portion). At its distal end, the tail is continuous with the ductus deferens. During ejaculation, peristaltic contractions of the smooth muscles lining the ducts propel the sperm and 5% of the seminal fluid into the ductus deferens.

Ductus Deferens (Vas Deferens or Seminal Duct) The ductus deferens is a tube about 18 inches long that carries spermatozoa from the epididymis of each testis to an ejaculatory duct during *emission*. It ascends along the posterior border of the epididymis, enters the pelvic cavity through the inguinal canal, and loops over the side and down the posterior surface of the urinary bladder. Before it enters the prostate gland, the ductus deferens is dilated and is called the *ampulla*. A seminal vesicle joins the duct at the distal end of the ampulla.

Ejaculatory Duct The distal end of the ampulla is continuous with a short tube about one inch long called the ejaculatory duct, which passes into the prostate gland and joins the prostatic urethra.

Urethra The urethra is a tube that extends from the urinary bladder to the tip of the penis. It is divided into three parts: the *prostatic urethra* passes through the prostate gland; the *membranous urethra* passes through the urogenital diaphragm; and the *spongy urethra* passes through the corpus spongiosum of the penis.

GLANDS

Seminal Vesicles The paired seminal vesicles are about two inches long. They lie posterior to and at the base of the urinary bladder. They secrete an alkaline, viscous fluid containing fructose, prostaglandins, and fibrinogen into the ejaculatory ducts. This fluid helps to neutralize the acidic environment in the female reproductive tract and provides nourishment for the sperm. It constitutes about 60% of the volume of semen.

Prostate Gland The prostate gland is a single, doughnut-shaped gland about the size of a chestnut that surrounds the superior portion of the urethra just inferior to the urinary bladder. It secretes a milky, slightly acidic fluid into the urethra through many prostatic ducts. The fluid contains citric acid and several enzymes (acid phosphatase, clotting enzymes, and fibrinolysin). It contributes to sperm motility and viability and constitutes about 25% of the volume of semen.

Bulbourethral Glands (Cowper's Glands) The paired bulbourethral glands are about the size of peas. They lie beneath the prostate gland on either side of the membranous urethra within the urogenital diaphragm; their ducts open into the spongy urethra. During sexual intercourse, they secrete 10% of the seminal fluid, which is alkaline and contains mucus.

DUCTS AND GLANDS

Lateral View

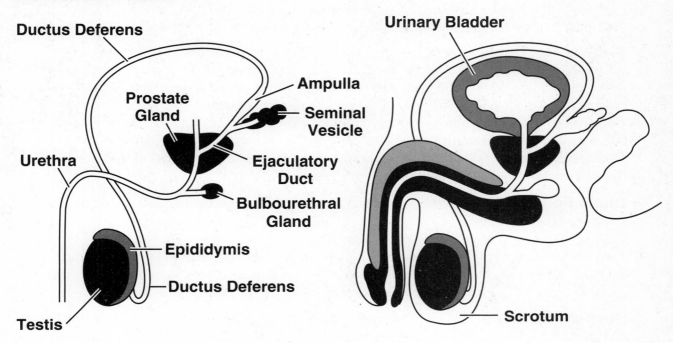

Ductus Deferens

Prostate
Gland

Ampulla

Seminal
Vesicle

Ejaculatory
Duct

Urethra

Bulbourethral
Gland

Epididymis

Ductus Deferens

Testis

Urinary Bladder

Scrotum

Front View

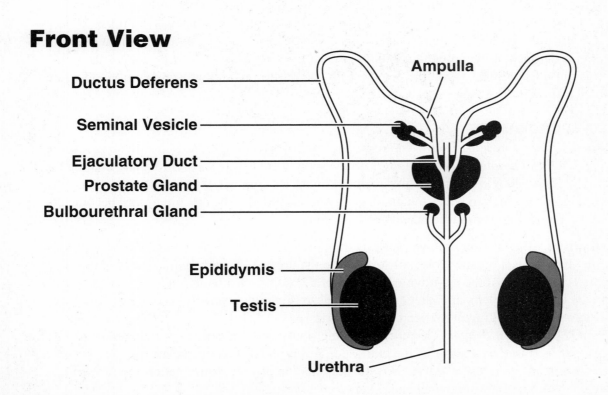

Ductus Deferens

Ampulla

Seminal Vesicle

Ejaculatory Duct

Prostate Gland

Bulbourethral Gland

Epididymis

Testis

Urethra

MALE REPRODUCTIVE SYSTEM / Penis

STRUCTURES

The penis is the male organ of copulation. It contains three cylindrical masses of spongy tissue that can become engorged with blood, causing erection. The enlarged and stiffened penis is inserted into the female vagina during sexual intercourse. It has three main parts: body, glans penis, and root.

Body of the Penis   The body is the free, pendulous part of the penis. It consists of three cylindrical masses of spongy erectile tissue. Two of these structures, the corpora cavernosa, form the upper (dorsal) two-thirds of the body; the other structure, the corpus spongiosum, forms the lower (ventral) third of the body. The body of the penis is covered by skin.

Corpora Cavernosa (singular: corpus cavernosum)   The corpora cavernosa of the penis are the two dorsolateral masses of erectile tissue.

Corpus Spongiosum   The corpus spongiosum is the smaller midventral mass of spongy erectile tissue; it contains the spongy urethra.

Glans Penis (*glandes* = acorn)   The glans penis is the distal end of the corpus spongiosum. It forms the tip of the penis.

Corona   The corona is the margin of the glans penis.

External Urethral Orifice   The external urethral orifice is the slitlike opening of the urethra.

Prepuce (Foreskin)   The prepuce or foreskin is the skin that covers the glans penis. It is often surgically removed by a procedure called *circumcision*.

Root of the Penis   The root of the penis is the attached portion. It consists of the crura, bulb, and the muscles associated with them.

Crura of Penis (singular: crus of penis)   The crura (*crura* = legs) of the penis are the separated and tapered portions of the corpora cavernosa. Each crus of the penis is attached to the ischial and inferior pubic rami and surrounded by the *ischiocavernosus muscle*. When they contract, these muscles force blood from the crura into the distal parts of the corpora cavernosa, increasing the stiffness of the penis. They also compress the *deep dorsal vein*, which impedes drainage.

Bulb of Penis   The bulb of the penis is the expanded base of the corpus spongiosum. It is attached to the inferior surface of the urogenital diaphragm and is enclosed by the *bulbospongiosus muscle*. When this muscle contracts, it compresses the bulb and the corpus spongiosum, emptying the urethra of residual urine and/or semen.

SEXUAL INTERCOURSE

Erection   When a male is stimulated erotically, arterioles leading to the penis dilate in response to *parasympathetic stimulation*. Blood flows into the spongy erectile tissues, filling and dilating the spaces. The bulbospongiosus and ischiocavernosus muscles contract, compressing the veins of the corpora cavernosa, which impedes the drainage of venous blood. The erectile tissues become engorged with blood; the penis stiffens and becomes erect.

Ejaculation   Ejaculation has two phases: emission and expulsion of semen.

Emission   Emission is the movement of semen into the urethra. *Sympathetic stimulation* causes peristaltic contractions of the epididymis, ductus deferens, and ejaculatory ducts, forcing spermatozoa into the urethra. Other sympathetic impulses cause rhythmic contractions of the seminal vesicles and prostate gland, resulting in the secretion of fluids.

Expulsion (Ejaculation Proper)   Expulsion is the propulsion of semen out of the urethra at the time of orgasm. It is caused by spasms of the bulbospongiosus and ischiocavernosus muscles in response to *parasympathetic stimulation*. *Orgasm* is the culmination of sexual stimulation; it involves a pleasureable feeling of physiological and psychological release.

MALE REPRODUCTIVE ORGANS
Sagittal Section

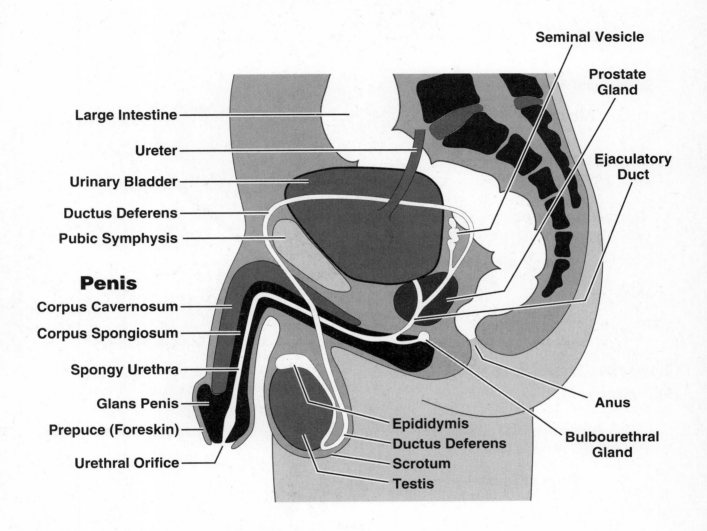

Seminal Vesicle

Prostate Gland

Ejaculatory Duct

Large Intestine

Ureter

Urinary Bladder

Ductus Deferens

Pubic Symphysis

Penis

Corpus Cavernosum

Corpus Spongiosum

Spongy Urethra

Glans Penis

Prepuce (Foreskin)

Urethral Orifice

Epididymis

Ductus Deferens

Scrotum

Testis

Anus

Bulbourethral Gland

PENIS

Cross Section

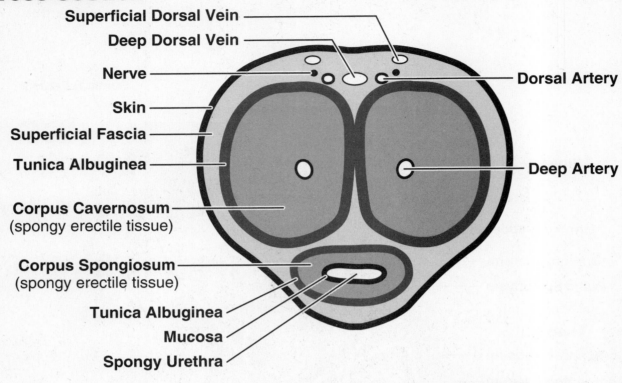

Superficial Dorsal Vein

Deep Dorsal Vein

Nerve

Skin

Superficial Fascia

Tunica Albuginea

Corpus Cavernosum
(spongy erectile tissue)

Corpus Spongiosum
(spongy erectile tissue)

Tunica Albuginea

Mucosa

Spongy Urethra

Dorsal Artery

Deep Artery

Coronal Section
(Skin removed)

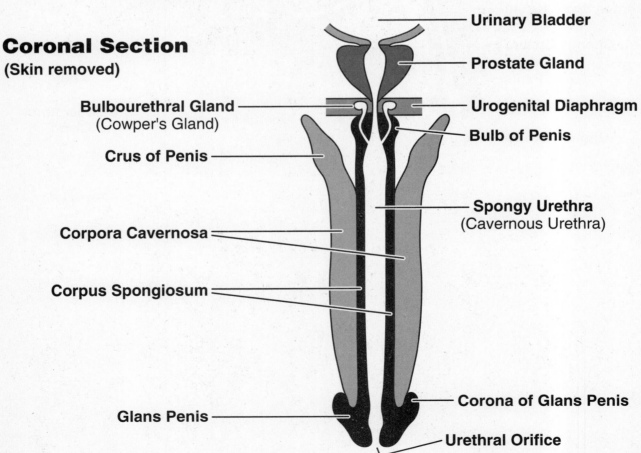

Bulbourethral Gland
(Cowper's Gland)

Crus of Penis

Corpora Cavernosa

Corpus Spongiosum

Glans Penis

Urinary Bladder

Prostate Gland

Urogenital Diaphragm

Bulb of Penis

Spongy Urethra
(Cavernous Urethra)

Corona of Glans Penis

Urethral Orifice

ERECTION

Reflex Pathway
Spongy erectile tissue fills with blood.

Input from the brain
inhibits or facilitates erection

Sensory
Nerve

Arteriole

Sacral Nerves
(S2 - S4)

Penis

Spongy
Erectile
Tissue

Motor
Nerve
(Parasympathetic)

Mechano-
receptor

Arterioles Dilate
(Veins constrict passively)

Penis
(cross-section)

Dorsal Artery

Deep Artery

Sacral Nerves
(S2 - S4)

2
3
4

Spongy Erectile
Tissue

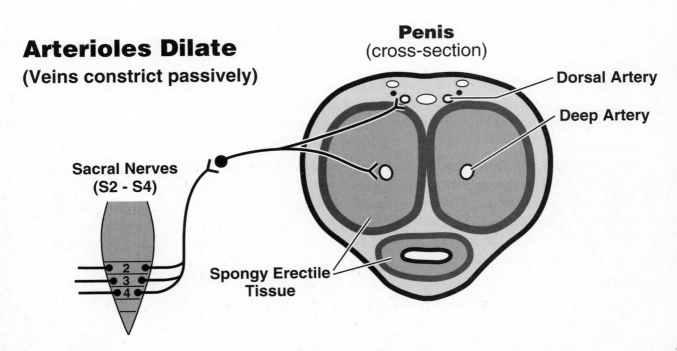

MALE REPRODUCTIVE SYSTEM / Semen

Semen   Semen is a mixture of sperm and the secretions of the seminal vesicles, prostate gland, and bulbourethral glands. The following outline summarizes the characteristics and components of semen.

CHARACTERISTICS

Volume   The average volume of semen in an ejaculation is 2.5–5 ml. A low volume might suggest an anatomical or functional defect or inflammation.

Color   Fluid from the prostate gland gives semen a milky appearance.

Sperm Count   The average ejaculation contains 50–150 million spermatozoa per milliliter. A male is likely to be infertile if the number of spermatozoa is below 20 million/ml. Sperm counts between 20 and 40 million/ml are borderline normal. The very large number of spermatozoa is necessary because only a tiny fraction ever reach the ovum (egg) in the uterine tubes (Fallopian tubes) of the female reproductive tract. Also, in order to penetrate an ovum, a sperm must release certain enzymes from the acrosome; one sperm does not produce enough of these enzymes to dissolve the barrier (zona pellucida) surrounding the ovum.

Motility   At least 60% of the spermatozoa in an ejaculation should show good forward motility within the first three hours after collecting the specimen.

pH   Semen has a slightly alkaline pH of 7.20–7.60. A rise in pH could indicate prostatitis.

Specific Gravity   Semen is denser than water; specific gravity is 1.028.

Morphology   No more than 20% of the spermatozoa should have abnormal shapes, such as a poorly formed head or tail.

COMPONENTS

Antibiotics
Seminalplasmin   Semen contains an antibiotic called seminalplasmin. It inhibits the growth of bacteria, which are present in semen and in the lower female reproductive tract.

Nutrients
Fructose   The fluid secreted by the seminal vesicles contains the sugar fructose, which provides sperm with an energy source. Mitochondria located in the middle piece of a spermatozoon use fructose to produce ATP, which is necessary for the movement of the tail.

Enzymes
Hyaluronidase and *Proteinase*   Spermatozoa secrete hyaluronidase and proteinases from their acrosomes. These enzymes digest the material covering the ovum (the zona pellucida).
Clotting Enzymes   Once in the vagina, semen coagulates rapidly (clotting enzymes secreted by the prostate gland act on fibrinogen produced by the seminal vesicles).
Fibrinolysin   Coagulated semen liquifies after 5–20 minutes. Fibrinolysin, produced by the prostate gland, dissolves the clot.

Buffers
Buffers, such as phosphate and bicarbonate, keep the pH of the semen relatively constant.

SEMEN

Characteristics

Volume	2.5 to 5 ml per ejaculation
Color	milky appearance (due to prostatic secretion)
Sperm Count	50 to 150 million sperm per ml
Motility	at least 60% active (show good forward motility)
pH	slightly alkaline (ranges between 7.20 and 7.60)
Specific Gravity	1.028 (denser than water)
Morphology	at least 80% normal (fewer than 20% abnormal forms)

Other Components

Antibiotics	seminalplasmin
Nutrients	fructose
Enzymes	hyaluronidase, proteinases, clotting enzymes, and fibrinolysin
Buffers	phosphate and bicarbonate

MALE REPRODUCTIVE SYSTEM / Hormonal Control

Male reproductive function is largely controlled by five hormones: (1) GnRH (gonadotropin-releasing hormone), (2) FSH (follicle-stimulating hormone), (3) LH (luteinizing hormone), (4) inhibin, and (5) testosterone.

GONADOTROPINS

At puberty (sometime between ages 10 and 14), there is an increase in the secretion of GnRH by the hypothalamus. There is a rhythmical nature to the secretion of this hormone: the neurons that secrete GnRH fire a burst of nerve impulses every two hours, and at these times GnRH is released. This hormone is secreted into the hypothalamo–pituitary portal vessels and carried to the anterior pituitary gland, where it stimulates the release of gonadotropins (FSH and LH). The target cells in the anterior pituitary gland will not respond to GnRH if the plasma concentration remains constant over time.

FSH *(Sustentacular Cell)* FSH stimulates sustentacular (Sertoli) cells in the seminiferous tubules. In response to FSH (and testosterone), the sustentacular cells secrete chemicals that stimulate spermatogenesis. They also secrete the hormone *inhibin*, which has a negative feedback effect on the anterior pituitary gland, inhibiting the secretion of FSH.

LH *(Interstitial Endocrinocyte)* LH stimulates interstitial endocrinocytes (interstitial cells of Leydig), which are located in the interstitial spaces between the seminiferous tubules. In response to LH, the interstitial endocrinocytes secrete the male sex hormone testosterone.

ANDROGENS

Male sex hormones are collectively called androgens. *Testosterone* is synthesized from cholesterol in the testes, and is the principal androgen. It also functions as a prohormone (hormone precursor) for another androgen, *dihydrotestosterone (DHT)*. The principal actions of androgens are outlined below.

Development Before birth, testosterone stimulates the male pattern of development of reproductive system ducts and the descent of the testes into the scrotum. DHT stimulates development of the external genitals (scrotum and penis). Androgens are also converted into estrogens that play a role in the development of certain regions of the brain.

Spermatogenesis Together with FSH, testosterone stimulates spermatogenesis.

Behavior Testosterone is responsible for the development of the sex drive (libido) at puberty, and it plays a role in the maintenance of the sex drive in the adult male.

Metabolism Androgens are anabolic hormones: they stimulate protein synthesis, which leads to heavier muscle and bone mass in males. They cause the cessation of bone growth by stimulating closure of the epiphyseal plate (near the end of a bone). They also increase the rate of metabolism and the production of red blood cells.

Secondary Sex Characteristics Male secondary sex characteristics are features that develop at puberty under the influence of androgens, but are not directly involved in sexual reproduction. Examples include muscular and skeletal growth that results in wide shoulders and narrow hips; characteristics of pubic, axillary, facial and chest hair; thickening of the skin; increased sebaceous gland secretion; and enlargement of the larynx (deepening of the voice).

MALE REPRODUCTIVE HORMONES

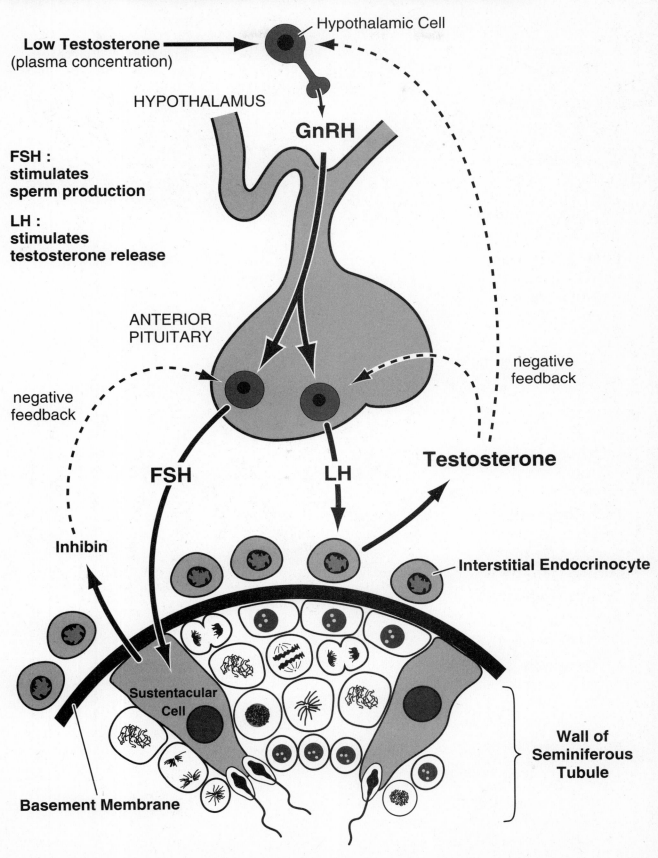

Hypothalamic Cell

Low Testosterone
(plasma concentration)

HYPOTHALAMUS

GnRH

FSH :
stimulates
sperm production

LH :
stimulates
testosterone release

ANTERIOR
PITUITARY

negative
feedback

negative
feedback

FSH

LH

Testosterone

Inhibin

Interstitial Endocrinocyte

Sustentacular
Cell

Wall of
Seminiferous
Tubule

Basement Membrane

23

2 Female Reproductive System

FEMALE REPRODUCTIVE SYSTEM / Overview

STRUCTURES

The female organs of reproduction include the ovaries, uterine tubes, uterus, vagina, vulva, and mammary glands.

Ovaries   The ovaries are the female *gonads* (gonad is general term for a gland that produces gametes and sex hormones). They are the primary sex organs of the female.

Uterine Tubes and Uterus   Each uterine tube (or Fallopian tube) is about four inches long, and extends laterally from the uterus to an ovary. The uterus (or womb) is a hollow organ located between the urinary bladder and the rectum. A fertilized ovum is transported through a uterine tube to the uterus, where it lodges (implants) in the uterine lining and develops into an embryo.

Vagina   The vagina is a tubular structure about four inches long that extends from the uterus to the exterior. It is the female organ of copulation (sexual intercourse) and serves as a passageway for menstrual flow and childbirth.

Vulva   The vulva (or pudendum) refers to the external genitalia of the female. It includes the mons pubis, labia majora, labia minora, clitoris, and vestibule.

Mammary Glands   The mammary glands are modified sudoriferous (sweat) glands that produce milk. They lie over the pectoralis major and serratus anterior muscles and are attached to them by a layer of connective tissue.

REPRODUCTIVE CYCLE

The female reproductive cycle (or menstrual cycle) lasts about 28 days and has four phases: menstrual phase, preovulatory phase, ovulation, and postovulatory phase. During each phase, significant events (controlled by hormones) occur in the ovaries and uterus. Each month a follicle matures in one ovary.

Menstrual Phase   In the ovary, in response to rising levels of FSH secreted by the anterior pituitary gland, about twenty primary follicles develop into secondary follicles. Due to low levels of estrogen and progesterone, the inner lining of the uterus sloughs off. Between 50 and 150 ml of blood, tissue fluid, mucus, and epithelial cells pass from the uterine cavity through the vagina to the exterior.

Preovulatory Phase   In the ovary, due to decreased levels of FSH, the less-developed secondary follicles degenerate. One dominant secondary follicle survives and develops into a mature follicle (vesicular ovarian follicle). In response to rising levels of estrogen, the endometrium thickens.

Ovulation   In the ovary, in response to a surge of LH secreted by the anterior pituitary gland, the mature follicle ruptures, and a secondary oocyte is propelled into a uterine tube. In response to high estrogen levels, the endometrium continues to thicken.

Postovulatory Phase   During the early part of this phase, under the influence of LH, the ruptured follicle develops into a new structure called the corpus luteum. The corpus luteum secretes estrogen and progesterone, which prepare the endometrium to receive a fertilized ovum. If fertilization and implantation do not occur, the corpus luteum degenerates, the levels of progesterone and estrogen decrease, and the endometrium begins to degenerate.

PREGNANCY

Pregnancy is a sequence of events that usually includes fertilization, implantation, embryonic development, and fetal development. It ends with birth (about 266 days after fertilization).

FEMALE REPRODUCTIVE ORGANS
Front View

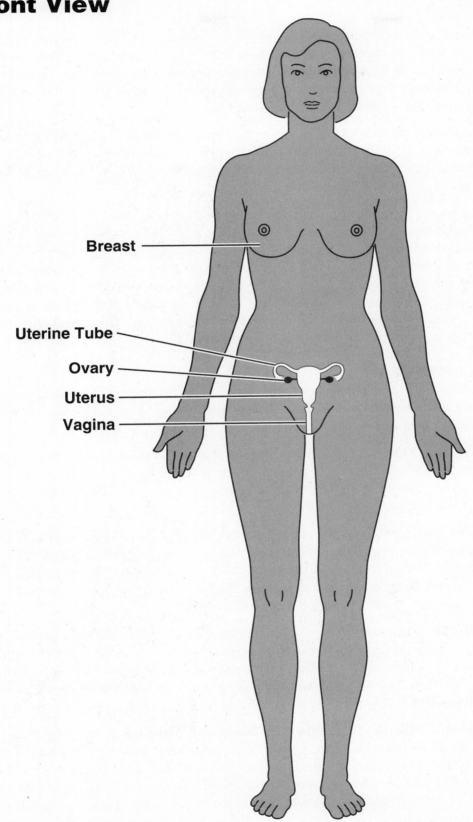

Breast

Uterine Tube

Ovary

Uterus

Vagina

FEMALE REPRODUCTIVE SYSTEM / Ovaries

STRUCTURES

The ovaries are paired almond-shaped structures about 1.5 inches long, 1.0 inch wide, and 0.5 inch thick. They have the same embryonic origin as the testes, and, like the testes, they produce gametes and sex hormones. They lie in the upper pelvic cavity, one on each side of the uterus. Each ovary has a *hilus*, a depressed area where blood vessels enter and leave. A double-layered fold of peritoneum called the *mesovarium* is attached to the hilus.

Ligaments Several ligaments hold the ovaries in position. The *broad ligament* of the uterus attaches to the anterior border of the ovary; the *ovarian ligament* attaches the inferior border of the ovary to the uterus; and the *suspensory ligament* attaches the superior border of the ovary to the lateral wall of the pelvis.

Histology

Germinal Epithelium The surface of the ovary is covered by a layer of simple squamous or cuboidal epithelium that is called the germinal epithelium.

Stroma The stroma is a general term for the tissue that forms the framework of an organ. Under the germinal epithelium, the stroma forms a layer of dense connective tissue called the *tunica albuginea*, which is responsible for the whitish color of the ovary. Beneath the tunica albuginea is a region of the stroma called the *cortex*; ovarian follicles are embedded in this region. The central region of the ovary consists of loose connective tissue and is called the *medulla*.

FOLLICLE DEVELOPMENT

In the 2nd month of the embryonic development of a female, primordial germ cells called *oogonia* begin to appear in the endoderm of the yolk sac. The oogonia migrate to the developing ovaries, where they proliferate (increase in number) by mitosis.

Primordial Follicle During fetal development (from the 3rd to the 7th month), oogonia grow and differentiate into *primary oocytes*. Each primary oocyte is surrounded by a single layer of *granulosa (follicular) cells*, forming a structure called a *primordial follicle*. At birth, there are more than 200,000 primordial follicles in each ovary.

Primary Follicle Each month, starting at *puberty* (age 10–14), several primordial follicles develop into primary follicles. A *primary follicle* consists of a *primary oocyte* surrounded by multiple layers of *granulosa (follicular) cells*. A thick coat called the *zona pellucida*, which consists of glycoproteins, forms between the oocyte and the granulosa cells. The tissue (stroma) immediately surrounding the follicle differentiates into a layer of *theca cells*.

Secondary Follicle At the beginning of each menstrual cycle, in response to rising levels of FSH, about 20 primary follicles begin to develop into *secondary follicles*. At this time, the primary oocyte completes meiosis I, forming a *secondary oocyte* and a small cell called the *first polar body*. The *granulosa (follicular) cells* surrounding the secondary oocyte continue to proliferate and secrete a fluid, forming a fluid-filled cavity called the *follicular cavity* or *antrum*.

Vesicular Ovarian Follicle (Graafian or Mature Follicle) Usually only one secondary oocyte completely matures, forming a *vesicular (Graafian or mature) follicle*. The other secondary follicles disintegrate, a process called *atresia*. The vesicular ovarian follicle has a structure called the *cumulus oophorus*, which is composed of granulosa cells that protrude into the follicular cavity (antrum). During ovulation, a vesicular ovarian follicle ruptures, ejecting a secondary oocyte into the open funnel-shaped end of the adjacent uterine tube. The granulosa (follicular) cells of the ruptured follicle form a new structure called the *corpus luteum*.

OVARY

Ovarian Cycle

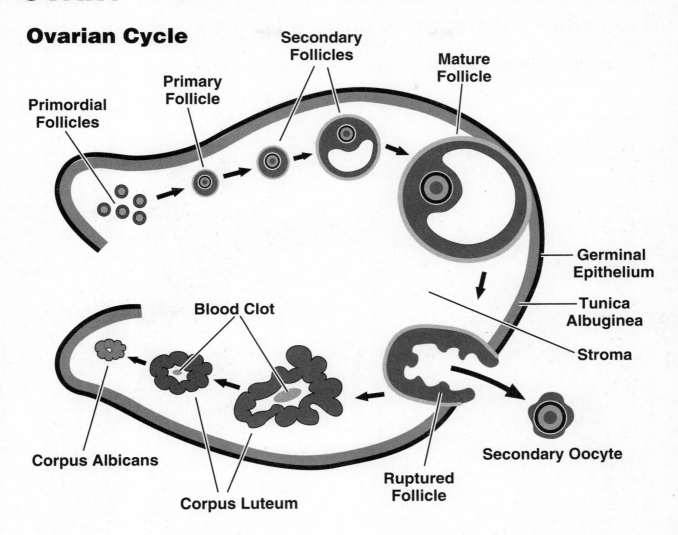

Primordial Follicles

Primary Follicle

Secondary Follicles

Mature Follicle

Germinal Epithelium

Tunica Albuginea

Stroma

Secondary Oocyte

Ruptured Follicle

Blood Clot

Corpus Luteum

Corpus Albicans

Vesicular Ovarian Follicle
(Graafian Follicle or Mature Follicle)

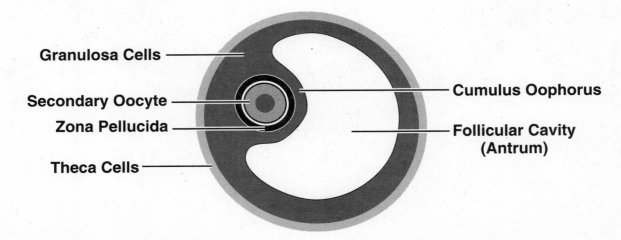

Granulosa Cells

Secondary Oocyte

Zona Pellucida

Theca Cells

Cumulus Oophorus

Follicular Cavity (Antrum)

VESICULAR OVARIAN FOLLICLE
also called a Graafian or Mature Follicle

A mature follicle contains a secondary oocyte in metaphase of meiosis II.

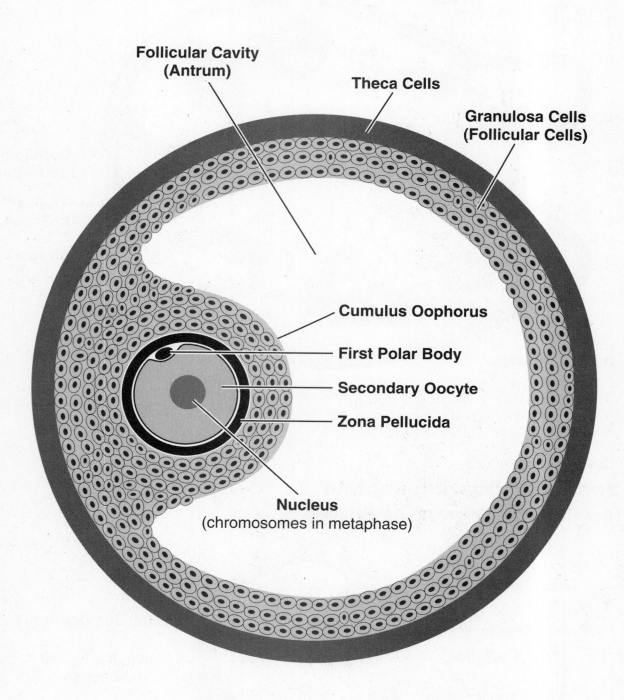

Follicular Cavity (Antrum)

Theca Cells

Granulosa Cells (Follicular Cells)

Cumulus Oophorus

First Polar Body

Secondary Oocyte

Zona Pellucida

Nucleus
(chromosomes in metaphase)

MATURE OVUM (EGG)

At the time of ovulation, a mature follicle ruptures, propelling a secondary oocyte from an ovary into a uterine tube.

Some of the granulosa (follicular) cells remain attached to the oocyte, forming a structure called the corona radiata.

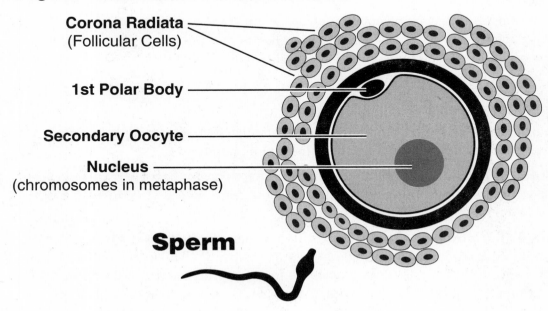

Corona Radiata
(Follicular Cells)

1st Polar Body

Secondary Oocyte

Nucleus
(chromosomes in metaphase)

Sperm

After fertilization, the secondary oocyte completes meiosis II, forming a small daughter cell (the second polar body) and a large daughter cell (the mature ovum).

The haploid nuclei of the sperm and the ovum are called pronuclei. The pronuclei fuse to form the diploid nucleus (segmentation nucleus) of the zygote.

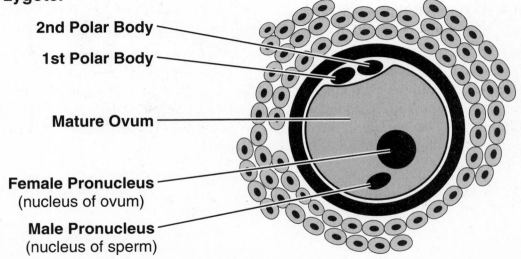

2nd Polar Body

1st Polar Body

Mature Ovum

Female Pronucleus
(nucleus of ovum)

Male Pronucleus
(nucleus of sperm)

FEMALE REPRODUCTIVE SYSTEM / Oogenesis

Oogenesis   The formation of ova (eggs) in the ovaries is called oogenesis. It is essentially the same as spermatogenesis, which occurs in the testes. The basic difference is that one spermatogonium produces four spermatozoa, while one oogonium produces only one ovum (and two small cells called polar bodies, which disintegrate).

MITOSIS OF OOGONIA

Early in the embryonic development of a female, some of the endoderm cells lining the yolk sac differentiate into primordial germ cells. These cells migrate to the developing ovaries and become oogonia (singular: oogonium). During early fetal development, the oogonia divide by mitosis, forming clones of oogonia.

MEIOSIS OF OOCYTES

In a female fetus, all of the oogonia grow and differentiate into primary oocytes. Both oogonia and primary oocytes have 46 chromosomes (the diploid number).

Meiosis I *(Prophase)*   In the fetus, all of the primary oocytes begin to divide by meiosis, but stop in the first stage of the process (prophase). These germ cells are said to be in a state of *meiotic arrest* until puberty.

Meiosis I *(Completion)*   At birth, each ovary contains about 200,000 primary oocytes. Each primary oocyte is surrounded by a single layer of granulosa (follicular) cells, forming a structure called a *primordial follicle*. No new oocytes are formed during the life of the female. (This is in contrast to a male, who continues to produce new spermatocytes throughout his life.)

At puberty, the ovaries become active. In response to the rising level of FSH that occurs at the start of each menstrual cycle, several primordial follicles develop into primary follicles. In a *primary follicle*, the oocyte is surrounded by several layers of granulosa (follicular) cells. At this time, meiosis I, which stopped during fetal development, continues to completion. The result is two cells, each with 23 chromosomes (the haploid number). The two daughter cells are of unequal size. The smaller cell is called the *first polar body*; the larger cell is called the *secondary oocyte*.

Meiosis II *(Metaphase)*   After completion of meiosis I, the secondary oocyte immediately begins meiosis II, but stops in metaphase. The granulosa (follicular) cells surrounding the secondary oocyte continue to proliferate. The follicle grows into a *secondary follicle*, containing a fluid-filled follicular cavity (antrum) and finally becomes a *mature follicle* just before ovulation.

Meiosis II *(Completion)*   At ovulation, the secondary oocyte (in metaphase of meiosis II) is discharged from the ovary into the uterine tube. If spermatozoa are present and fertilization occurs, meiosis II continues to completion. Two unequal daughter cells result: the smaller cell is called the *second polar body*; the larger cell is called the *ovum* (or mature egg). The nucleus of the ovum fuses with the nucleus of the spermatozoon, forming a diploid nucleus (46 chromosomes). The cell with the diploid nucleus is called a *zygote*.

OOGENESIS
Production of an Ovum by Meiosis

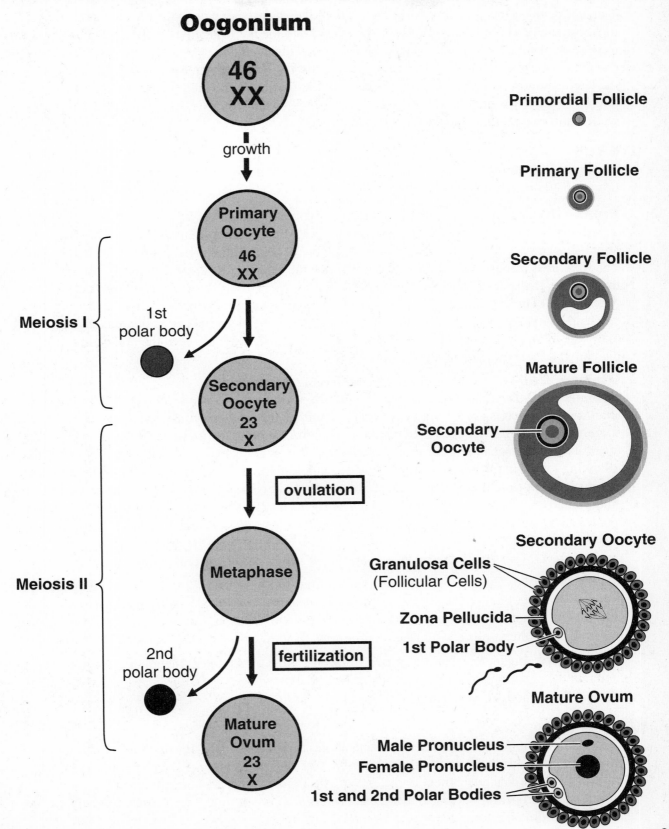

Oogonium

46 XX

growth

Primary Oocyte 46 XX

Meiosis I

1st polar body

Secondary Oocyte 23 X

Meiosis II

ovulation

Metaphase

2nd polar body

fertilization

Mature Ovum 23 X

Primordial Follicle

Primary Follicle

Secondary Follicle

Mature Follicle

Secondary Oocyte

Secondary Oocyte

Granulosa Cells (Follicular Cells)

Zona Pellucida

1st Polar Body

Mature Ovum

Male Pronucleus
Female Pronucleus
1st and 2nd Polar Bodies

FEMALE REPRODUCTIVE SYSTEM / Uterus and Vagina

UTERINE TUBES (Fallopian Tubes or Oviducts)

The uterine tubes extend laterally on each side of the uterus. Each is about 4 inches long and 0.5 inches in diameter; each opens at its proximal end into the uterus, and at its distal end into the peritoneal cavity near an ovary. The open, funnel-shaped distal end of each tube, called the *infundibulum*, ends in a fringe of fingerlike projections called *fimbriae* (singular: fimbria); one fimbria is attached to the lateral end of the ovary. The longest and widest portion of the tube (about two-thirds of its length) is called the *ampulla*; this is where fertilization usually occurs. The short, narrow, thick-walled portion that joins the uterus is called the *isthmus*.

UTERUS

The uterus (or womb) is a hollow organ with the shape of an inverted pear. It is located between the urinary bladder and the rectum. Before the first pregnancy it is about 3 inches long.

Parts   The uterus consists of two major parts: the body and the cervix. The *body* is the expanded superior two-thirds of the uterus; the *cervix*, or neck, is the inferior cylindrical portion. The superior dome-shaped portion of the body located above the entrance of the uterine tubes is called the *fundus*. The *isthmus* is a constricted portion about 0.5 inch long that marks the junction between the body and the cervix. The space inside the body is called the *uterine cavity*; the space inside the cervix is called the *cervical canal*. The *internal os* is the narrow passageway between the uterine cavity and the cervical cavity; the *external os* is the narrow passageway between the cervix and the vagina. Normally the uterus is in a position called *anteflexion*; there is a bend between the body and cervix, so the body projects over the urinary bladder.

Uterine Wall   The wall of the uterus consists of three layers.
Endometrium   The inner layer. The endometrium is divided into two layers: (1) the *stratum functionalis*, which is shed during menstruation and (2) the *stratum basalis*, which gives rise to a new stratum functionalis after each menstruation. If implantation of the blastocyst occurs, the stratum functionalis becomes modified, and is called the *decidua*; all of the decidua is shed with the placenta following birth. In the pregnant uterus, the decidua is divided into three portions: (1) the *decidua basalis* is the portion that underlies the embryo; (2) the *decidua capsularis* is the portion between the embryo and the uterine cavity; and (3) the *decidua parietalis* is the remaining modified endometrium that lines the uterus.
Myometrium   The middle layer. It consists of three layers of smooth muscle fibers.
Perimetrium (Serosa)   The outer layer. This layer is part of the visceral peritoneum.

Blood Supply   The uterus is supplied by branches of the *internal iliac artery* called the *uterine arteries*. Branches called the *arcuate arteries* are arranged in a circular fashion and give off *radial arteries* that penetrate the myometrium. The radial arteries branch, forming *straight arterioles* that end in the stratum basalis and *spiral arterioles* that penetrate the stratum functionalis.

Ligaments   Ligaments that are either extensions of the parietal peritoneum or fibromuscular cords maintain the position of the uterus. They include the *broad ligaments*, *cardinal ligaments* (lateral cervical ligaments), *uterosacral ligaments*, and *round ligaments*.

VAGINA

The vagina is a tubular, fibromuscular organ about four inches long. It is the female organ of copulation. It is located between the urinary bladder and the rectum. A recess called the *fornix* surrounds the vaginal attachment to the cervix. A thin fold of mucous membrane at the vaginal orifice (vaginal opening) is called the *hymen*; it forms a border around the orifice, partially closing it. It is usually torn and destroyed by the first sexual intercourse.

FEMALE REPRODUCTIVE ORGANS
Sagittal Section

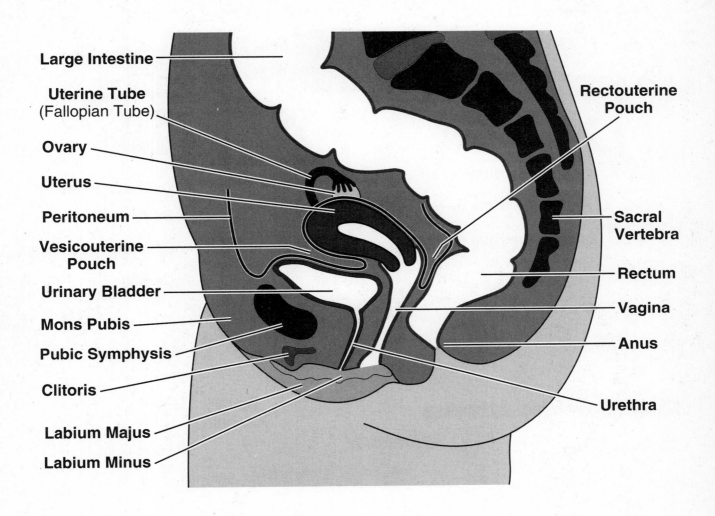

Large Intestine

Uterine Tube
(Fallopian Tube)

Ovary

Uterus

Peritoneum

Vesicouterine
Pouch

Urinary Bladder

Mons Pubis

Pubic Symphysis

Clitoris

Labium Majus

Labium Minus

Rectouterine
Pouch

Sacral
Vertebra

Rectum

Vagina

Anus

Urethra

UTERUS

Uterus and Associated Structures

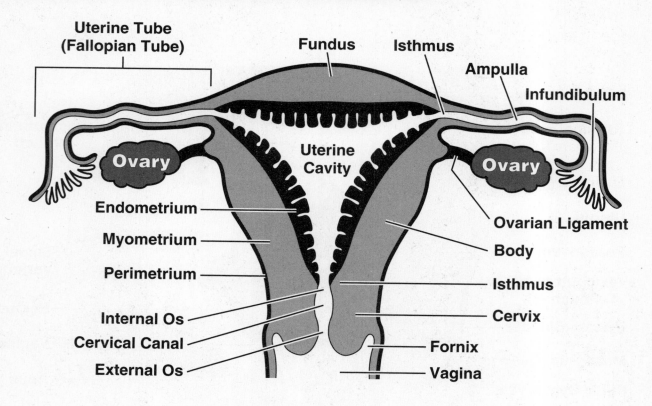

Uterine Tube (Fallopian Tube)

Fundus

Isthmus

Ampulla

Infundibulum

Ovary

Uterine Cavity

Ovary

Endometrium

Myometrium

Perimetrium

Internal Os

Cervical Canal

External Os

Ovarian Ligament

Body

Isthmus

Cervix

Fornix

Vagina

Lining of the Uterus

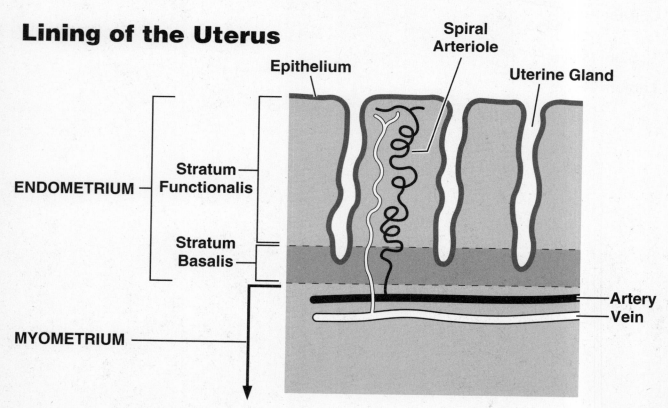

Epithelium

Spiral Arteriole

Uterine Gland

ENDOMETRIUM

Stratum Functionalis

Stratum Basalis

MYOMETRIUM

Artery

Vein

PREGNANT UTERUS

Decidua

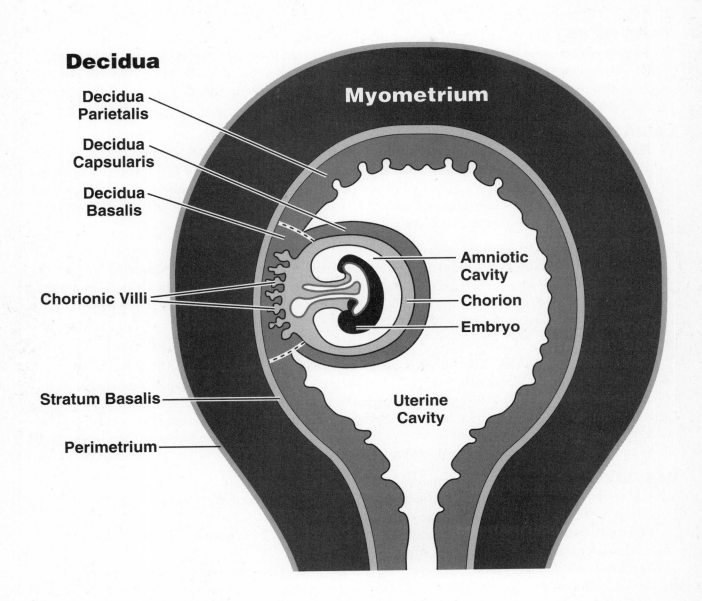

Decidua Parietalis

Decidua Capsularis

Decidua Basalis

Myometrium

Chorionic Villi

Amniotic Cavity

Chorion

Embryo

Stratum Basalis

Uterine Cavity

Perimetrium

FEMALE REPRODUCTIVE SYSTEM / Vulva

Vulva (Pudendum)   (*volvere* = to wrap around)   The term vulva (or pudendum) refers to the external genitalia of the female. It consists of five parts: mons pubis, labia majora, labia minora, clitoris, and vestibule.

MONS PUBIS   (*mons* = mountain; *pubis* = of the pubic bone)
The mon pubis is a rounded elevation located anterior to the pubic symphysis. It consists of a pad of fatty connective tissue. At puberty, the amount of fat increases and the mons pubis becomes covered by coarse pubic hairs. After menopause, the amount of fat and pubic hair decreases. The mons pubis cushions the pubic bone during sexual intercourse.

LABIA MAJORA   (*labia* = lips; *majora* = large)
Homologous to the Scrotum   The labia majora are homologous to the male scrotum.
The labia majora (singular: labium majus) are two symmetrical folds of skin filled with subcutaneous fat and covered by pubic hair. Each fold passes posteriorly from the mons pubis to about 2.5 cm from the anus. They contain an abundance of sebaceous (oil) and sudoriferous (sweat) glands. The labia majora protect the urethral and vaginal orifices.

LABIA MINORA   (*labia* = lips; *minora* = small)
The labia minora (singular: labium minus) are thin, delicate folds of hairless skin located between the labia majora, enclosing the vestibule of the vagina. They contain sebaceous and sweat glands, but no fat. Just superior to the clitoris, the labia minora meet to form a fold of skin called the *prepuce* (foreskin), which covers the body of the clitoris.

CLITORIS
Homologous to the Penis   The clitoris is homologous to the male penis. The clitoris is a small cylindrical mass of erectile tissue about 3 cm in length. Like the penis, it is capable of enlargement upon tactile stimulation. It is highly sensitive and important in the sexual arousal of the female. It contains two corpora cavernosa, but no corpus spongiosum. Like the penis, the clitoris consists of a root, body, and glans. The *root* and *body* of the clitoris are covered by the prepuce (foreskin) formed by the labia minora. The *glans* is the exposed portion of the clitoris.

VESTIBULE   (*vestibulum* = antechamber)
The vestibule is the cleft (space) between the labia minora. The urethra, vagina, and ducts of the greater vestibular glands open into the vestibule.
External Urethral Orifice   The opening to the urethra is about 2 cm posterior to the clitoris and immediately anterior to the vaginal orifice.
Paraurethral Glands (Skene's Glands)   The paraurethral glands, which are homologous to the prostate gland in the male, secrete mucus. The ducts of these glands open on each side of the external urethral orifice.
Vaginal Orifice   The relatively large opening to the vagina is located posterior to the much smaller external urethral orifice. A thin fold of mucous membrane called the *hymen* surrounds the vaginal orifice.
Bulb of the Vestibule   The bulb of the vestibule is homologous to the corpus spongiosum and bulb of the penis; it consists of two elongated masses of erectile tissue about 3 cm in length on either side of the vaginal orifice. During sexual arousal it becomes engorged with blood, narrowing the vaginal orifice, which places pressure on the penis during intercourse.
Greater Vestibular Glands (Bartholin's Glands)   The greater vestibular glands are homologous to the bulbourethral glands of the male. They open by ducts into a groove between the hymen and the labia minora. They secrete mucus that supplements lubrication during sexual intercourse.

VULVA
Pudendum or External Genitalia

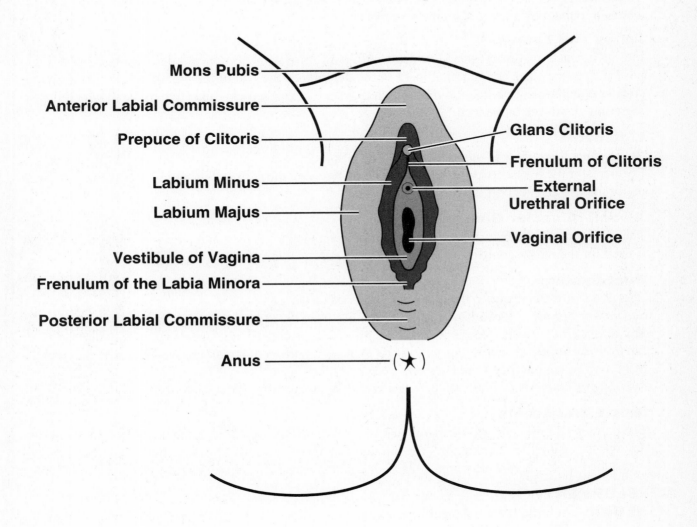

Mons Pubis

Anterior Labial Commissure

Prepuce of Clitoris

Labium Minus

Labium Majus

Vestibule of Vagina

Frenulum of the Labia Minora

Posterior Labial Commissure

Anus

Glans Clitoris

Frenulum of Clitoris

External Urethral Orifice

Vaginal Orifice

Mammary Glands   The mammary glands are modified sudoriferous (sweat) glands that are specialized to produce milk.

STRUCTURES

The mammary glands lie over the pectoralis major and serratus anterior muscles of the thorax and are attached to them by a layer of connective tissue.

Lobes and Lobules

Internally, each mammary gland consists of 15 to 20 compartments called *lobes*, separated by adipose (fat) tissue. The amount of adipose tissue determines the size of the breasts. Each lobe contains smaller compartments called *lobules*. The lobules are composed of connective tissue in which milk-secreting glands are embedded.

Ligaments

Suspensory Ligaments (Cooper's Ligaments)   Strands of connective tissue called the suspensory ligaments of the breasts (Cooper's ligaments) run between the skin and deep fascia of the pectoralis major muscle and support the breasts.

Alveoli (Alveolar Glands)

The milk-secreting glands are arranged in grapelike clusters and are called *alveoli* (the same term that is used for the microscopic air spaces in the lungs) or *alveolar glands*.

Duct System

The alveoli are connected to the exterior by a series of ducts.
Secondary Tubule   Secondary tubules carry milk from the alveoli to mammary ducts.
Mammary Duct   A mammary duct carries milk from secondary tubules to a lactiferous sinus.
Lactiferous Sinus   A lactiferous sinus is an expanded portion of a mammary duct near the nipple. Milk may be temporarily stored here.
Lactiferous Duct   A lactiferous duct carries milk from a lactiferous sinus to the exterior.

Nipple and Areola

The pigmented projection of the mammary gland is called the *nipple*. Lactiferous ducts carry milk through the nipples to the exterior. The circular pigmented area of skin surrounding the nipple is called the *areola*. It appears rough because it contains modified sebaceous (oil) glands.

DEVELOPMENT

At Birth   At birth, both male and female mammary glands are undeveloped and appear as slight elevations on the chest.

Puberty   At puberty, under the influence of estrogen and progesterone, the female breasts begin to develop. The duct system matures, extensive fat deposition occurs, and the areola and nipple grow and become pigmented.

LACTATION

Lactation refers to the secretion and ejection of milk by the mammary glands.
Secretion *(Prolactin)*   Even though prolactin levels increase during pregnancy, the presence of estrogen and progesterone inhibit prolactin from being effective. After delivery, the levels of estrogen and progesterone decrease, the inhibition is removed, and the mammary glands secrete milk.
Ejection *(Oxytocin)*   The sucking action of the infant initiates nerve impulses to the hypothalmus that stimulate the secretion of oxytocin (OT) by the posterior pituitary. Oxytocin induces *myoepithelial cells* surrounding the walls of the alveoli to contract. This compresses the alveoli and ejects milk into the ducts, where it can be suckled.

MAMMARY GLAND

Sagittal Section

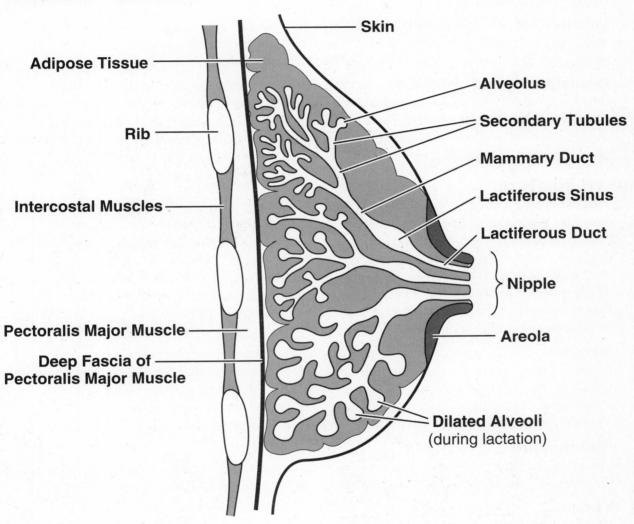

Skin

Adipose Tissue

Alveolus

Secondary Tubules

Rib

Mammary Duct

Lactiferous Sinus

Intercostal Muscles

Lactiferous Duct

Nipple

Pectoralis Major Muscle

Areola

Deep Fascia of
Pectoralis Major Muscle

Dilated Alveoli
(during lactation)

Duct System

Lobule
(connective tissue)

Alveolus

Secondary Tubules

Mammary Duct

Lactiferous Duct

Lactiferous Sinus

THE FEMALE SEXUAL ACT

Erection Psychic and tactile stimulation triggers a reflex. Parasympathetic impulses from the sacral spinal cord travel to the external genitalia, especially the clitoris. The clitoris becomes engorged with blood and erect.

Lubrication Parasympathetic impulses also travel to the vagina, resulting in the secretion of mucus from the epithelium of the cervical mucosa and the greater vestibular glands (Bartholin's glands) that open into a groove between the hymen and the labia minora.

Orgasm (Climax) When tactile stimulation of the genitalia reaches maximum intensity, reflexes are initiated that cause the female orgasm (climax). Sympathetic impulses cause the *perineal muscles* to contract rhythmically. There is an increase in muscle tension throughout the body, engorgement of the clitoris and breasts, an increase in heart rate and breathing, and rhythmic contractions of the uterus. Intense pleasurable sensations are followed by general relaxation.

BIRTH CONTROL

Hormones

Norplant Six capsules containing *progestin* (a chemical similar to progesterone) are surgically implanted under the skin of the arm. Over five years, they slowly release progestin, which inhibits ovulation and thickens the cervical mucus.

Oral Contraceptive (OC or "The Pill") The most commonly used pills contain a high concentration of progesterone and a low concentration of estrogen, causing a negative feedback effect on the hypothalamus and the anterior pituitary gland. The resulting low levels of FSH and LH usually prevent the development of a follicle.

Barriers Barrier methods prevent spermatozoa from entering the uterine cavity.

Cervical Cap A cervical cap is a thimble-shaped device made of latex that fits over the cervix.

Condom A condom is a nonporous, elastic (latex) covering placed over the penis.

Diaphragm A diaphragm is a rubber, dome-shaped device that fits over the cervix.

Vaginal Pouch A vaginal pouch is a polyurethane sheath that fits over the cervix of the uterus.

Spermicides

Spermicides are sperm-killing chemicals that are inserted into the vagina. Contraceptive sponges are effective for 24 hours. Creams, douches, foams, jellies, and suppositories are effective for 1 hour.

Timing

Rhythm Method Sexual intercourse is avoided for about 7 days (just before and after ovulation).

Sympto–thermal Method The signs of ovulation are used to determine the period of abstinence.

Sterilization

Vasectomy (in males) A portion of each ductus deferens is removed, so sperm cannot be ejaculated. Spermatozoa produced in the testes degenerate and are phagocytized.

Tubal Ligation (in females) A portion of each uterine tube is removed, so the spermatozoa cannot reach the secondary oocyte, and the oocyte cannot pass into the uterus.

Intrauterine Device (IUD) An intrauterine device is a small object made of plastic, copper, or stainless steel that is inserted into the cavity of the uterus. It causes changes in the uterine lining that block implantation of a fertilized ovum.

Withdrawal (Coitus Interruptus) The penis is withdrawn from the vagina before ejaculation occurs.

Abortion Surgical or drug-induced removal of the embryo.

BIRTH CONTROL

Methods	Examples	Comments
Hormones	Norplant Oral Contraceptive ("The Pill")	Estrogen and progesterone prevent follicle development and ovulation.
Barriers	Cervical Cap Condom Diaphragm Vaginal Pouch	Sperm are prevented from entering the uterine cavity. Male condoms protect against sexually transmitted diseases.
Spermicides	Contraceptive Sponge Creams Douches Foams Jellies Suppositories	These methods depend upon sperm-killing chemicals. The contraceptive sponge releases spermicide for up to 24 hours.
Timing	Rhythm Method Sympto–thermal Method	The avoidance of sexual intercourse for about 7 days (while a viable ovum is in the uterine tube).
Sterilization	Vasectomy (male) Tubal Ligation (female)	The severing of each ductus deferens in the male and both uterine tubes in the female.
Intrauterine Device (IUD)		An object placed in the uterine cavity prevents implantation.
Withdrawal (Coitus Interruptus)		The penis is withdrawn from the vagina before ejaculation occurs.
Abortion		Surgical or drug-induced removal of the embryo.

3 Female Reproductive Cycle

FEMALE REPRODUCTIVE CYCLE / Overview

FEMALE REPRODUCTIVE CYCLE

The female reproductive cycle, or menstrual cycle, encompasses the ovarian cycle, the uterine cycle, and the cyclical changes in the breasts and cervix that occur each month. It lasts about 28 days (varies from 24 to 35 days). It may be divided into four phases:

Menstrual Phase The first 5 days; the uterine lining is shed.
Preovulatory Phase Days 6–13; a follicle matures.
Ovulation Day 14; the mature follicle ruptures, ejecting an oocyte into a uterine tube.
Postovulatory Phase Days 15–28; the corpus luteum secretes estrogen and progesterone.

OVARIAN CYCLE

The ovarian cycle is a series of events associated with the maturation of an ovum.
Follicle Development It generally takes about 20 days (the last 6 days of the previous cycle and the first 14 days of the current cycle) for a *primordial follicle* to develop into a *mature follicle* (vesicular ovarian follicle). During this time a primary oocyte completes meiosis I and becomes a secondary oocyte; just before ovulation, the secondary oocyte reaches metaphase of meiosis II.

Follicular Phase The follicular phase includes the menstrual phase and preovulatory phase (days 1 – 13). Follicles are growing and developing at this time.

Luteal Phase The postovulatory phase (days 15 – 28) is also called the luteal phase, because the corpus luteum is functioning at this time.

UTERINE CYCLE

The uterine cycle is a series of changes in the endometrium of the uterus. Each month, the endometrium is prepared for the arrival of a fertilized ovum that will develop in the uterus until birth. If fertilization does not occur, the stratum functionalis portion of the endometrium is shed.

Menstrual Phase The menstrual phase (days 1–5) is the first phase of the uterine cycle. It is the period of time during which the uterine lining (the stratum functionalis) is being sloughed off.

Proliferative Phase The preovulatory phase (days 6–13) is also called the proliferative phase, because the cells of the uterine lining are increasing in number (proliferating).

Secretory Phase The postovulatory phase (days 15–28) is also called the secretory phase, because glands in the endometrium secrete glycogen and other substances.

REPRODUCTIVE HORMONES

The principal events of the reproductive cycle are controlled by hormones.

GnRH The hypothalamus secretes gonadotropin-releasing hormone (GnRH), which stimulates the anterior pituitary gland to secrete follicle-stimulating hormone (FSH) and luteinizing hormone (LH).

Gonadotropins (FSH and LH) FSH stimulates the initial development of the ovarian follicles and the secretion of estrogen by the follicles. LH stimulates further development of the ovarian follicles, ovulation, and the secretion of estrogen and progesterone by the corpus luteum.

Estrogen and Progesterone Estrogen and progesterone are secreted by the ovaries and the corpus luteum. They have many different functions, which are discussed later in this chapter.

Inhibin Inhibin is secreted by the corpus luteum. It has a negative feedback effect on the hypothalamus and the anterior pituitary gland, inhibiting the secretion of GnRH and FSH.

FEMALE REPRODUCTIVE CYCLE

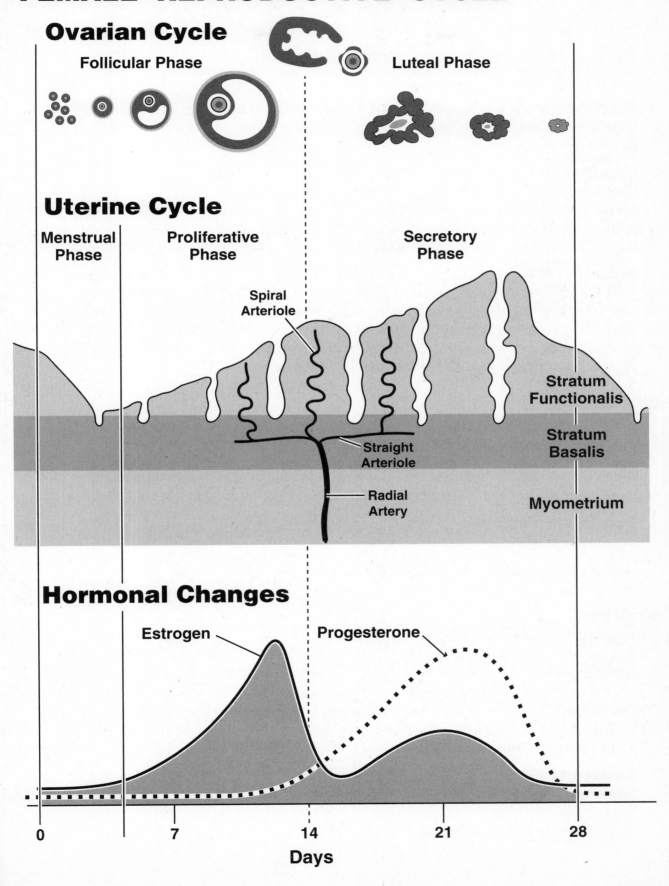

Ovarian Cycle

Follicular Phase

Luteal Phase

Uterine Cycle

Menstrual Phase

Proliferative Phase

Secretory Phase

Spiral Arteriole

Straight Arteriole

Radial Artery

Stratum Functionalis

Stratum Basalis

Myometrium

Hormonal Changes

Estrogen

Progesterone

0   7   14   21   28

Days

FEMALE REPRODUCTIVE CYCLE / Menstrual Phase
Days 1 – 5

Menstrual Phase   The menstrual phase, which lasts about five days, is also called *menstruation* or *menses*. By convention, the first day of menstruation marks the first day of a new cycle.

HYPOTHALAMUS AND ANTERIOR PITUITARY GLAND

During the menstrual phase, GnRH is secreted by the hypothalamus and FSH is secreted by the anterior pituitary gland.

Hypothalamus

GnRH   In response to low levels of estrogen, neurosecretory cells in the hypothalamus release gonadotropin-releasing hormone (GnRH), which diffuses into a capillary network called the *primary plexus*. From the primary plexus, the blood drains into the *hypophyseal portal veins* that pass down the stalk of the pituitary gland (the *infundibulum*) to the anterior pituitary gland.

Anterior Pituitary

FSH   In the anterior pituitary gland, the hypophyseal portal veins form a capillary network called the *secondary plexus*. GnRH diffuses out of the secondary plexus and acts on its target cells (*gonadotrophs*) in the anterior pituitary gland. FSH, released by the gonadotrophs, diffuses into the secondary plexus and is carried to the *anterior hypophyseal veins*, which carry blood out of the anterior pituitary gland into the general circulation.

OVARY
Primary Follicles

At about day 25 of the previous cycle, a number of primordial follicles begin to develop into primary follicles. A clear glycoprotein layer called the *zona pellucida* forms between the secondary oocyte and the granulosa cells. During the early part of each menstrual phase, in response to rising levels of FSH, about twenty primary follicles develop into secondary follicles.

Secondary Follicles

 A secondary follicle consists of a *secondary oocyte* surrounded by several layers of *granulosa (follicular) cells*. The granulosa cells secrete estrogen and follicular fluid (forms the *follicular cavity* or *antrum*). As the granulosa cells proliferate, the secretion of estrogen increases.

UTERUS
Stratum Functionalis

The discharge that occurs during menstruation is due to the declining levels of estrogen and progesterone during the final days of the previous cycle. Low levels of estrogen and progesterone causes the *spiral arterioles* in the inner lining of the uterus (the *stratum funcionalis*) to constrict and rupture. When the spiral arterioles constrict, the blood supply to the stratum functionalis is cut off and the endometrial cells in this portion of the uterine lining die. As a result, the entire stratum functionalis sloughs off, leaving the *stratum basalis* as the inner lining.

Menstrual Flow

Menstrual flow consists of 50 to 150 ml of blood, tissue fluid, mucus, and epithelial cells derived from the endometrium (lining of the uterus). It passes from the uterine cavity to the cervix and through the vagina to the exterior.

MENSTRUAL PHASE (days 1 to 5)

Hypothalamus : GnRH released.

Anterior Pituitary : FSH released.

Ovary : Primordial follicles develop into primary follicles, then into secondary follicles.

Primordial follicles start to develop during the previous cycle (about day 25).

Granulosa (follicular) cells secrete low levels of estrogen.

Granulosa cells secrete follicular fluid that fills the follicular cavity (antrum)

Uterus : Inner lining of endometrium (stratum functionalis) sloughs off.

Spiral arterioles constrict (due to low levels of estrogen and progesterone).

Cells of the stratum functionalis die (due to lack of nourishment).

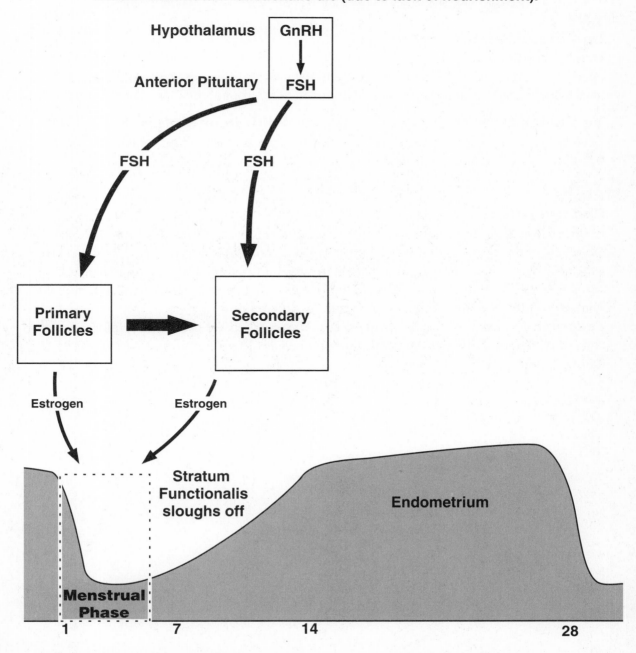

Preovulatory Phase The preovulatory phase preceeds ovulation. It is more variable than the other phases, lasting between six and thirteen days in a 28-day cycle.

HYPOTHALAMUS AND ANTERIOR PITUITARY GLAND

During the early part of the preovulatory phase, *moderate levels* of estrogen cause a *negative* feedback inhibition of FSH secretion. In the late part of the preovulatory phase, *high levels* of estrogen have a *positive* feedback effect on the secretion of FSH. Early in the preovulatory phase, FSH is the dominant gonadotropin secreted by the anterior pituitary. Close to the time of ovulation, however, LH is secreted in increasing quantities.

OVARY
Dominant Secondary Follicle

During the early part of the preovulatory phase, decreased FSH levels cause the less well-developed secondary follicles to stop growing and degenerate, a process called *atresia*.   One dominant follicle survives and secretes enough estrogen to promote its own growth and development.

Vesicular Ovarian Follicle (Graafian Follicle or Mature Follicle)

The one dominant secondary follicle matures into a vesicular ovarian follicle (also called a Graafian follicle or a mature follicle).

UTERUS
Endometrium

Estrogen, the dominant hormone secreted by the developing vesicular ovarian follicle, stimulates the repair of the endometrium. Cells of the *stratum basalis* undergo mitosis and produce a new *stratum functionalis*. As the endometrium thickens, the short, straight endometrial glands develop and the spiral arterioles coil and lengthen as they penetrate the stratum functionalis. The thickness of the endometrium nearly doubles to about 5 mm.

Proliferative Phase The preovulatory phase is also called the proliferative phase, because the cells of the endometrium are increasing in number (proliferating), resulting in a thickening of the uterine lining.

PREOVULATORY PHASE (days 6 to 13)

Hypothalamus : GnRH released.

Anterior Pituitary : FSH released.

Moderate levels of estrogen (early part of phase) have a negative feedback effect.
High levels of estrogen (late part of phase) have a positive feedback effect.

Ovary : Most secondary follicles degenerate (due to decreased FSH secretion).

One dominant secondary follicle matures into a vesicular ovarian follicle.

Granulosa (follicular) cells secrete estrogen.

Uterus : Endometrium thickens; stimulated by estrogen.

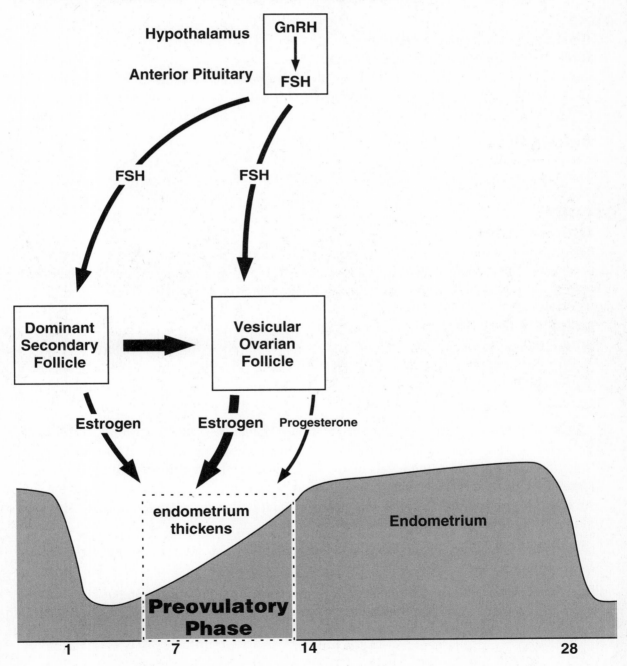

FEMALE REPRODUCTIVE CYCLE / Ovulation
Day 14

Ovulation Ovulation is the rupture of a vesicular ovarian follicle with the discharge of a secondary oocyte into a uterine tube. It usually occurs on day fourteen of a 28-day cycle.

HYPOTHALAMUS AND ANTERIOR PITUITARY GLAND
Just before ovulation, the *high level* of estrogen that developed during the latter part of the preovulatory phase exerts a *positive feedback* effect on the hypothalamus and anterior pituitary gland, increasing the secretion of GnRH and LH. The sudden surge of LH triggers ovulation. (This positive feedback effect does not occur if progesterone is also present.)

OVARY
Vesicular Ovarian Follicle
Just before ovulation occurs, the secondary oocyte in the mature follicle reaches metaphase of meiosis II. During ovulation, the secondary oocyte remains surrounded by the zona pellucida and a covering of granulosa cells (follicular cells). These granulosa cells are collectively called the the *corona radiata*.

Corpus Hemorrhagicum
After ovulation, the vesicular ovarian follicle collapses to become the *corpus hemorrhagicum*. The collapsed follicle contains a blood clot that is eventually absorbed by granulosa cells.

UTERUS
Uterine Tube
The fimbriae of the uterine tubes drape over the ovaries and become active near the time of ovulation. Movements of the fimbriae and the action of cilia lining the uterine tube create currents in the peritoneal fluid that carry the secondary oocyte into the uterine tube.

SIGNS OF OVULATION
(1) Basal Temperature One sign of ovulation is an increase in basal temperature (body temperature at rest). An increase in temperature (usually between 0.4 and 0.6°F) occurs about 14 days after the start of the last menstrual cycle; it is due to increasing levels of progesterone. The 24 hours following this rise in temperature is the best time to become pregnant.

(2) Cervical Mucus Another sign of ovulation is the amount and consistency of cervical mucus. Secretion of cervical mucus is regulated by estrogen and progesterone. At mid-cycle, near the time of ovulation, increasing levels of estrogen cause secretory cells of the cervix to produce large amounts of cervical mucus. As ovulation approaches, the mucus becomes clear and very stretchy. If grasped with forceps, the mucus may stretch as far as 15 cm (6 in.). This type of mucus indicates the time of greatest fertility.

(3) Cervix The cervix also exhibits signs of ovulation. The external os opens, the cervix rises, and becomes softer.

(4) Mittelschmerz Some women also experience a pain in the area of one or both ovaries around the time of ovulation. Such pain is called mittelschmerz, meaning "pain in the middle," and may last from several hours to a day or two.

OVULATION (day 14)

Hypothalamus : GnRH released; stimulated by high levels of estrogen.

Anterior Pituitary : LH released in large quantities (called the LH surge).

Ovary : LH surge triggers ovulation.
Vesicular ovarian follicle ruptures, releasing the secondary oocyte.

Uterus : Endometrium thickens; stimulated by high levels of estrogen.

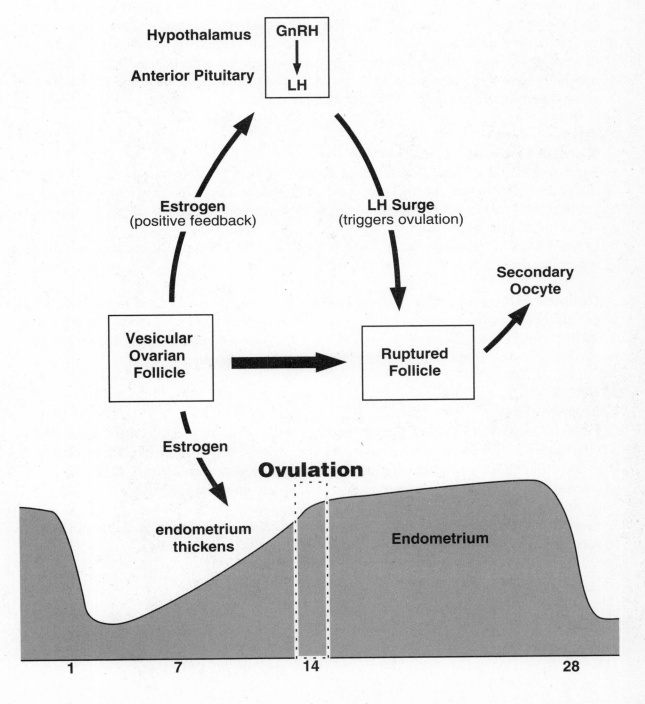

Postovulatory Phase The postovulatory phase follows ovulation. It is the most constant in duration, lasting 14 days (day 15 to 28) in a 28-day cycle. It is the period of time between ovulation and the onset of the next menstruation.

HYPOTHALAMUS AND ANTERIOR PITUITARY GLAND

After ovulation, LH secretion stimulates the development of the corpus luteum. If fertilization and implantation do not occur, the rising levels of estrogen and progesterone (secreted by the corpus luteum) have a *negative* feedback effect on the hypothalamus and anterior pituitary gland, inhibiting the secretion of GnRH and LH. Consequently, the corpus luteum degenerates, and the decreasing levels of estrogen and progesterone have a *positive* feedback effect on the hypothalamus and anterior pituitary gland. This promotes the secretion of GnRH and FSH, initiating another menstrual phase and a new reproductive cycle.

OVARY
Corpus Luteum

After ovulation, LH secretion stimulates the development of the corpus luteum. The granulosa (follicular) cells enlarge, change character, and form the corpus luteum. Corpus luteum means yellow body (*corpus* = body; *luteus* = yellow). Stimulated by LH, the corpus luteum secretes estrogen and progesterone.

Luteal Phase The postovulatory phase is also called the luteal phase, because the corpus luteum is functioning at this time.

Corpus Albicans
If fertilization and implantation do not occur, the rising levels of estrogen and progesterone (secreted by the corpus luteum) have a *negative* feedback effect that inhibits GnRH and LH secretion. As LH level declines, the corpus luteum degenerates and becomes the corpus albicans, or white body (*corpus* = body; *albus* = white).

UTERUS
Endometrium

Progesterone produced by the corpus luteum is responsible for preparing the endometrium (uterine lining) to receive a fertilized ovum. Preparatory activities include the growth of the endometrial glands and spiral arterioles, thickening of the endometrium, and an increase in the amount of tissue fluid. These preparatory changes are maximal about one week after ovulation, corresponding to the time when a fertilized ovum is most likely to arrive.

Secretory Phase The postovulatory phase is also called the secretory phase, because of the secretory activity of the endometrial glands (which secrete glycogen).

POSTOVULATORY PHASE (days 15 to 28)

Hypothalamus : GnRH released.

Anterior Pituitary : LH and FSH released.
    High levels of estrogen and progesterone inhibit the secretion of LH.
    Low levels of estrogen and progesterone stimulate the secretion of FSH.

Ovary : Under the influence of LH, granulosa cells are converted into the corpus luteum.

    The corpus luteum secretes estrogen and progesterone.

    As LH decreases, the corpus luteum becomes the corpus albicans
    (if fertilization has not occurred).

Uterus : Progesterone prepares the endometrium to receive a fertilized ovum.

    Decreasing levels of progesterone cause degeneration of the endometrium
    and initiate a new mentrual phase.

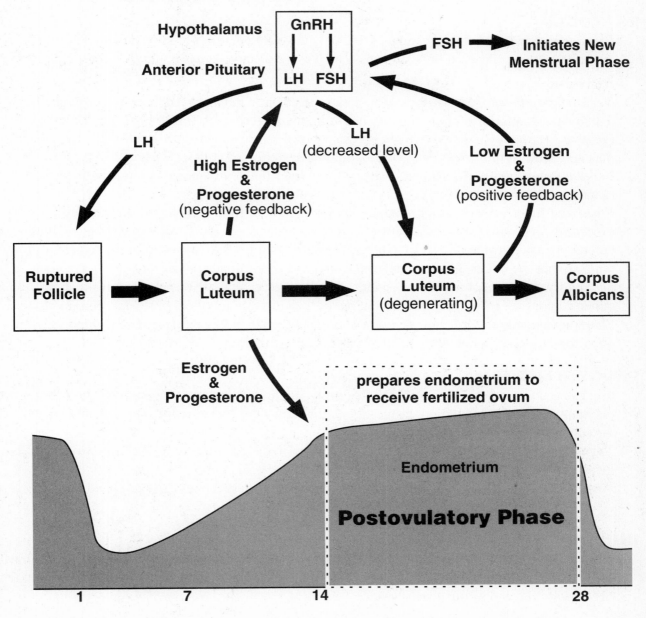

FEMALE REPRODUCTIVE CYCLE / Hormonal Control

GONADOTROPIN – RELEASING HORMONE (GnRH)

The hypothalamus secretes gonadotropin-releasing hormone (GnRH), which stimulates the anterior pituitary gland to secrete follicle-stimulating hormone (FSH) and luteinizing hormone (LH).

GONADOTROPINS (FSH and LH)

FSH During the early and middle parts of the preovulatory phase, FSH stimulates the granulosa cells (follicular cells) to proliferate and secrete estrogen.

LH During the late preovulatory phase, LH stimulates the theca cells (which surround the granulosa cells) to proliferate and secrete androgens, which are absorbed by nearby granulosa cells and converted into estrogen. At this time, high concentrations of estrogen cause an LH surge that stimulates ovulation and the formation of the corpus luteum. During the postovulatory phase, low levels of LH stimulate the corpus luteum to secrete estrogen and progesterone.

ESTROGEN

There are at least six different estrogens, but only three are present in significant quantities (beta-estradiol, estrone, and estriol). "Estrogen" is used as a collective term for all types of estrogens.

Actions

Negative Feedback *Moderate* levels of estrogen exert a *negative* feedback effect on the hypothalamus and anterior pituitary gland, inhibiting the secretion of GnRH, FSH, and LH.
Positive Feedback *High* levels of estrogen exert a *positive* feedback effect on the hypothalamus and anterior pituitary gland, stimulating the secretion of GnRH, FSH, and LH.
Female Reproductive Structures Estrogen promotes the development and maintenence of female reproductive structures (especially the lining of the uterus).
Fluid and Electrolyte Balance Estrogen helps to control fluid and electrolyte balance.
Protein Anabolism Estrogen stimulates protein synthesis (anabolism); it is synergistic with human growth hormone (hGH). (Synergistic means that the two hormones complement each other so that the target cells respond to the sum of the hormones involved.)
Secondary Sex Characteristics Female secondary sex characteristics are features that develop at puberty under the influence of estrogen, but are not directly involved in sexual reproduction. Examples include fat distribution in the breasts, abdomen, mons pubis, and hips; high voice pitch; broad pelvis; smooth skin texture; and hair distribution.

PROGESTERONE

Progesterone is secreted primarily by the corpus luteum. It prepares the endometrium for implantation. After implantation, progesterone maintains the endometrium and prepares the breasts to secrete milk.
Negative Feedback *High* levels of progesterone (in the presence of estrogen) have a *negative* feedback effect, inhibiting the secretion of GnRH, FSH, and LH.
Positive Feedback *Low* levels of progesterone (in the presence of estrogen) have a *positive* feedback effect, stimulating the secretion of GnRH, FSH, and LH.

INHIBIN

Inhibin is secreted by the corpus luteum. It has a negative feedback effect on the hypothalamus and the anterior pituitary gland, inhibiting the secretion of GnRH and FSH (and to a lesser extent LH) toward the end of the uterine cycle.

FEMALE REPRODUCTIVE HORMONES

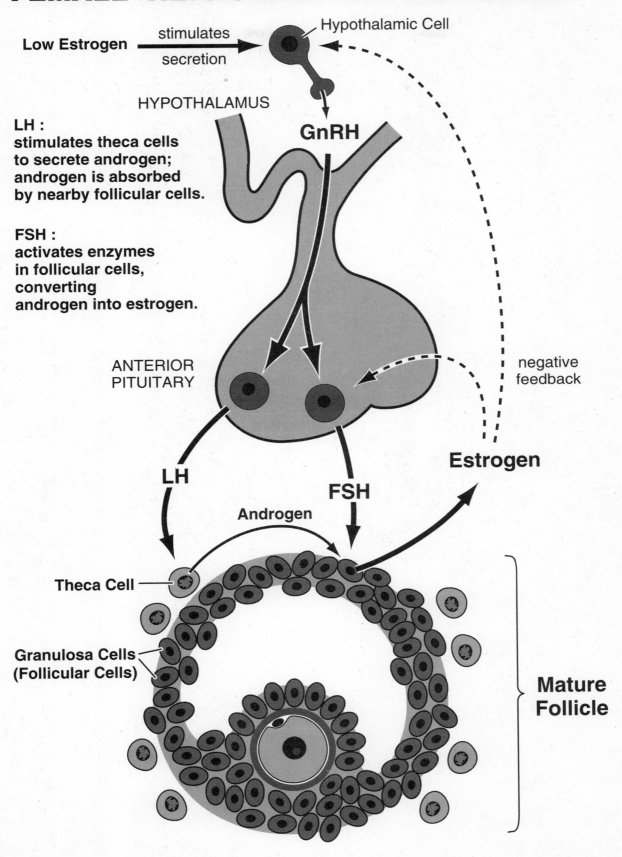

Low Estrogen — stimulates secretion → Hypothalamic Cell

HYPOTHALAMUS

GnRH

LH :
stimulates theca cells
to secrete androgen;
androgen is absorbed
by nearby follicular cells.

FSH :
activates enzymes
in follicular cells,
converting
androgen into estrogen.

ANTERIOR
PITUITARY

negative feedback

Estrogen

LH

FSH

Androgen

Theca Cell

Granulosa Cells
(Follicular Cells)

Mature
Follicle

4 Development

DEVELOPMENT / Overview

Developmental Anatomy   Developmental anatomy is the study of the sequence of events from the fetilization of a secondary oocyte to the formation of an adult organism.

WEEK ONE : CLEAVAGE

Fertilization   During fertilization, the genetic material (DNA) from a spermatozoon merges with the genetic material from a secondary oocyte, forming a diploid nucleus called a segmentation nucleus. The cell is now called a *mature ovum* or *zygote*.

Cleavage   Cleavage means repeated cell divisions without growth. Cleavage occurs as the dividing ovum passes through the uterine tube (Fallopian tube) toward the uterus. After about 36 hours, the zygote divides into two cells; after two days there are four cells; after four days there is a solid ball of cells called a *morula*; after five days the ball of cells develops a fluid-filled cavity and is called a *blastocyst*, which contains a specialized cluster of cells called the *inner cell mass*.

Implantation   About the sixth day after fertilization, the blastocyst attaches to the lining of the uterus (the endometrium). The outer cells, called the *trophoblast*, differentiate into two layers: the *cytotrophoblast* and the *syncytiotrophoblast*. The syncytiotrophoblast secretes enzymes that liquefy the endometrial cells, enabling the blastocyst to penetrate the uterine lining.

WEEK TWO : THE BLASTOCYST

During the second week, the blastocyst develops into an embryo.

Blastocyst   By the seventh day, the inner cell mass has differentiated into two primary germ layers, the *ectoderm* and the *endoderm*; the ectoderm forms a fluid-filled space called the amniotic cavity. By the twelfth day, the endoderm has formed a cavity called the *yolk sac*, which creates another space called the *extraembryonic coelom* between the yolk sac and the cytotrophoblast. The third type of primary germ cell, *mesoderm* cells, start to appear in the extraembryonic coelom.

Embryonic Disc   By the end of the second week (the fourteenth day), a layer of mesoderm has formed between a layer of ectoderm and endoderm, forming a trilaminar (three-layered) *embryonic disc*. From this time until the end of the eighth week, the developing organism is called an *embryo*.

EMBRYONIC DEVELOPMENT

Three major events occur during the embryonic period of development: (1) the *primary germ layers* differentiate, forming all the organs and tissues of the body; (2) *embryonic membranes* form; and (3) the *placenta* forms. The ectoderm forms the nervous system and the skin; the mesoderm forms bones, muscles, and blood; the endoderm forms the epithelial linings of the gastrointestinal and respiratory tracts. There are four embryonic membranes: *yolk sac*, *amnion*, *chorion*, and *allantois*. The placenta is a structure that allows for the exchange of materials between the blood of the mother and the blood of the embryo or fetus. It consists of the *chorion* of the embryo and the *decidua basalis* of the endometrium

FETAL DEVELOPMENT   3rd Month – end of the 9th Month

During the fetal period of development, all of the organs and tissues established by the primary germ layers grow rapidly and the fetus takes on a human appearance.

DEVELOPMENT

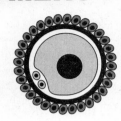

Zygote
(fertilized ovum)

Blastocyst
(5 days)
a hollow ball of cells

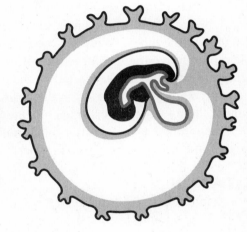

Embryo
(3 weeks)

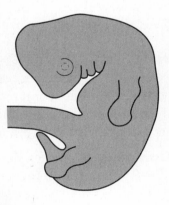

Embryo
(5 weeks)

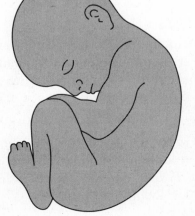

Fetus
(8 months)

DEVELOPMENT / Fertilization

TIME AND LOCATION

Of the 500 million spermatozoa that are introduced into the vagina during sexual intercourse, less than 1% reach the secondary oocyte in the uterine tube. Fertilization usually occurs in the uterine tube about 12 to 24 hours after ovulation. Secondary oocytes survive for only 12 to 24 hours following ovulation, while spermatozoa live up to 72 hours within the female reproductive tract. So, in order to have a spermatozoon and an oocyte that are both alive, sexual intercourse must occur no more than 72 hours before ovulation and no more than 24 hours following ovulation.

SPERM AND OOCYTE MOVEMENT

The secondary oocyte is moved through the uterine tube toward the uterus by peristaltic contractions and the action of ciliated epithelium that lines the uterine tubes. During sexual intercourse, semen is usually deposited in the vagina near the cervix. Several factors contribute to the movement of sperm toward the uterine tubes. Whiplike movements of the tail propel the sperm through the fluids in the female reproductive tract; contractions of the uterus stimulated by prostaglandins in the semen are thought to help; a chemical secreted by the oocyte attracts sperm; an enzyme called *acrosin*, which is produced by the acrosome (a sac in the head of the sperm), stimulates sperm motility and migration; and, under the influence of estrogen, the uterus and cervix produce a watery secretion that promotes sperm transport and survival (after ovulation, high progesterone concentrations cause the secretion of a viscous fluid that is unfavorable for sperm transport).

CAPACITATION

Capacitation refers to the functional changes that the spermatozoa undergo in the female reproductive tract that allow them to fertilize a secondary oocyte. During this process, which takes about 10 hours, the membrane around the acrosome becomes fragile, so that several enzymes (hyaluronidase, acrosin, and neuraminidase) can be secreted by the acrosome. These enzymes dissolve the corona radiata (granulosa cells) and the zona pellucida, so the sperm can penetrate the secondary oocyte.

PENETRATION OF THE OOCYTE

Syngamy   Normally, only one spermatozoon penetrates and enters a secondary oocyte, an event called syngamy. The tail of the sperm remains outside the oocyte, and the head develops into a structure called the *male pronucleus*. Calcium ions, released inside the oocyte, promote changes that block the entrance of other sperm, preventing *polyspermy* (fertilization by more than one sperm).

Meiosis II Completed   Once a spermatozoon has entered a secondary oocyte, the oocyte completes meiosis II; a large *ovum* (mature egg) and a second polar body are formed. The nucleus of the ovum develops into a *female pronucleus*.

FUSION OF THE PRONUCLEI

Zygote   The haploid female pronucleus fuses with the haploid male pronucleus, forming a diploid (2n) *segmentation nucleus*. The segmentation nucleus contains 23 chromosomes from the male pronucleus and 23 chromosomes from the female pronucleus. The fertilized ovum containing the diploid segmentation nucleus is called a *zygote*.

Twins

Dizygotic Twins (Fraternal Twins)   Dizygotic twins are produced from the independent release of two ova and the subsequent fertilization of each by different spermatozoa.
Monozygotic Twins (Identical Twins)   Monozygotic twins develop from a single fertilized ovum that splits at an early stage in development.

FERTILIZATION

Secondary Oocyte and Sperm

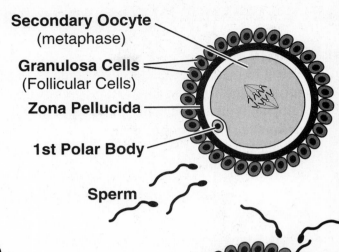

Secondary Oocyte (metaphase)

Granulosa Cells (Follicular Cells)

Zona Pellucida

1st Polar Body

Sperm

Penetration of the Oocyte

One sperm moves between the granulosa cells and binds to species-specific receptors on the zona pellucida.

With the aid of acrosomal enzymes, the sperm dissolves and penetrates the zona pellucida.

The head of the sperm fuses with oocyte plasma membrane.

Contractile elements in the oocyte draw in the head of the sperm, usually leaving the tail outside the oocyte.

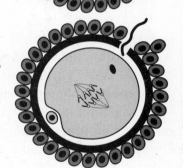

Fusion of the Pronuclei

After penetration, the oocyte completes meiosis II, forming an ovum and a 2nd polar body.

The nucleus in the ovum and the nucleus in the head of the sperm are called pronuclei.

The pronuclei fuse, forming a diploid nucleus called the segmentation nucleus.

The diploid cell is now called a zygote.

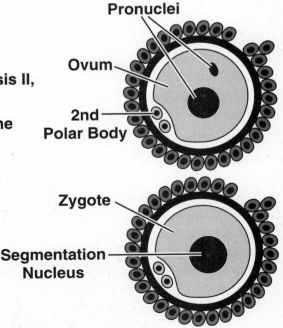

Pronuclei

Ovum

2nd Polar Body

Zygote

Segmentation Nucleus

DEVELOPMENT / Cleavage and Implantation

CLEAVAGE

The term *cleavage* means repeated cell divisions without growth. After fertilization, the zygote rapidly divides, forming about 50 progressively smaller cells in about five days. The size of the developing organism remains the same, since it is contained within the zona pellucida.

Blastomeres (*blast* = germ, sprout) The progressively smaller cells produced by cleavage are called blastomeres.

2-Cell Stage *(36 hours after fertilization)*

The first cleavage is completed about 36 hours after fertilization, and each succeeding division takes slightly less time.

4-Cell Stage *(2 days after fertilization)*

By the second day after fertilization, the second cleavage is completed.

16-Cell Stage *(3 days after fertilization)*

By the end of the third day, there are 16 cells.

Morula *(4 days after fertilization)*

Successive cleavages produce a solid mass of cells, still surrounded by the zona pellucida, called the morula (*morula* = mulberry). The morula is about the same size as the original zygote.

Blastocyst *(5 days after fertilization)*

About five days after fertilization, the dense cluster of cells has developed into a hollow ball of cells with a fluid-filled cavity. The structure is called a *blastocyst* and the cavity is called a *blastocoele*. The blastocyst passes from the uterine tube into the uterine cavity.

Trophoblast (*troph* = nourish) The outer covering of cells surrounding a blastocyst is called the trophoblast. Ultimately, the trophoblast forms part of the placenta.

Inner Cell Mass (Embryoblast) A mass of cells inside the trophoblast is called the *inner cell mass*. Part of the inner cell mass develops into the embryo. At this time, the zona pellucida disintegrates. The blastocyst receives nourishment from glycogen-rich secretions of endometrial glands, sometimes called *uterine milk*.

IMPLANTATION *(6 days after fertilization)*

About 6 days after fertilization, the blastocyst attaches to the endometrium (uterine lining), a process called implantation. The blastocyst usually implants on the posterior wall of the fundus or body of the uterus. The blastocyst is oriented so that the inner cell mass is toward the endometrium.

Trophoblast

Just before implantation, the trophoblast (the outer cells of the blastocyst) differentiates into two layers in the region of contact between the blastocyst and endometrium: the syncytiotrophoblast and the cytotrophoblast.

Syncytiotrophoblast (*synctium* = multinucleate mass) This layer contains no cell boundaries. During implantation, it secretes enzymes that enable the blastocyst to penetrate the uterine lining. The enzymes digest and liquefy the endometrial cells.

Cytotrophoblast (*cyto* = cell) This layer is composed of distinct cells, which form a continuous layer inside the syncytiotrophoblast.

CLEAVAGE AND IMPLANTATION

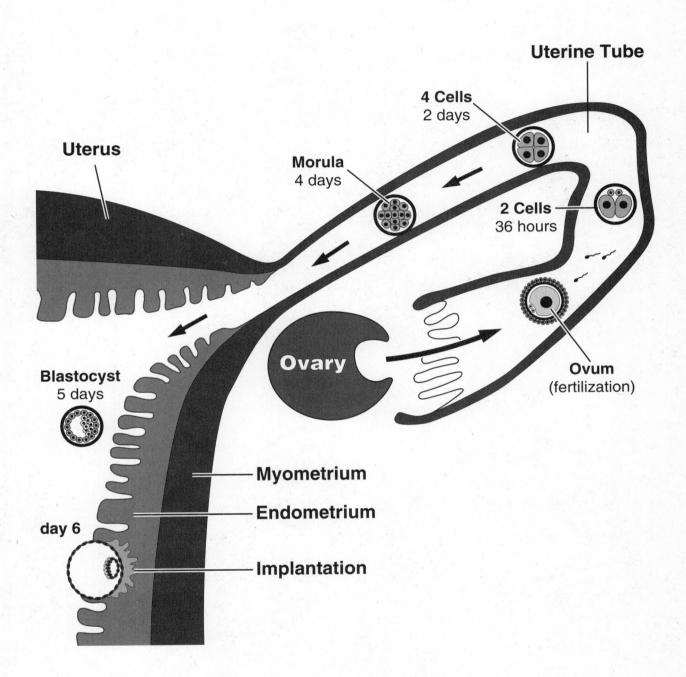

Uterine Tube

4 Cells
2 days

Morula
4 days

2 Cells
36 hours

Uterus

Ovary

Ovum
(fertilization)

Blastocyst
5 days

Myometrium

Endometrium

day 6

Implantation

CLEAVAGE

Cleavage and the formation of the morula and blastocyst.

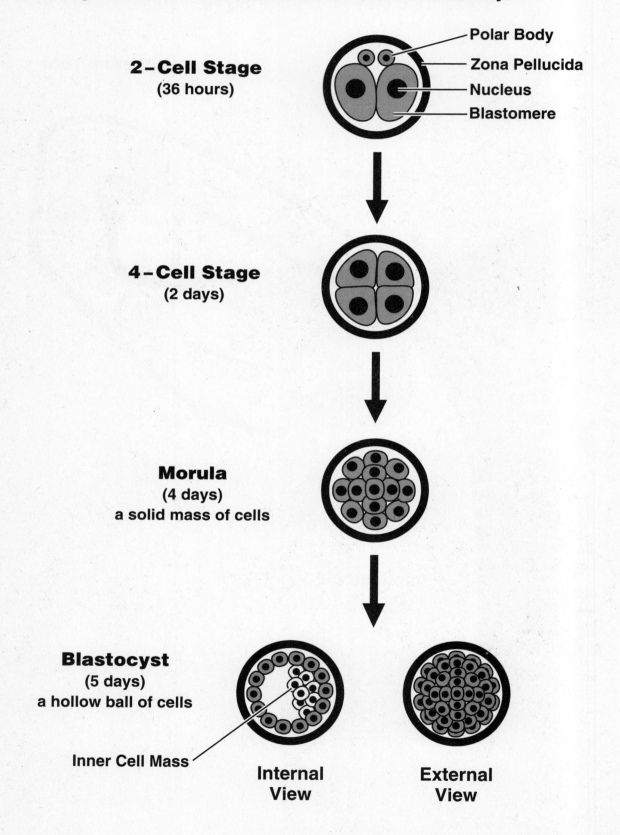

2–Cell Stage
(36 hours)

Polar Body
Zona Pellucida
Nucleus
Blastomere

4–Cell Stage
(2 days)

Morula
(4 days)
a solid mass of cells

Blastocyst
(5 days)
a hollow ball of cells

Inner Cell Mass

Internal
View

External
View

IMPLANTATION

Day 5

Blastocyst is free in the uterine cavity.

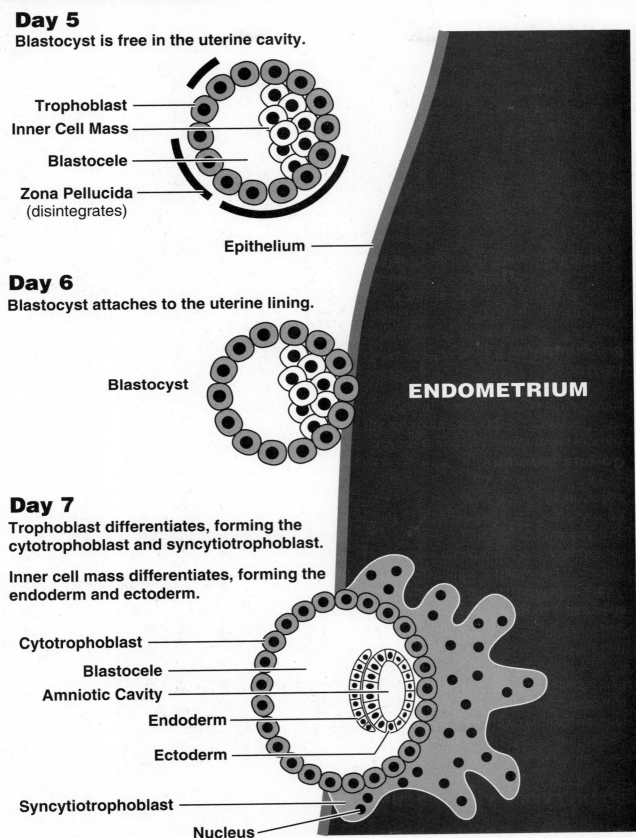

Trophoblast

Inner Cell Mass

Blastocele

Zona Pellucida
(disintegrates)

Epithelium

Day 6

Blastocyst attaches to the uterine lining.

Blastocyst

ENDOMETRIUM

Day 7

Trophoblast differentiates, forming the cytotrophoblast and syncytiotrophoblast.

Inner cell mass differentiates, forming the endoderm and ectoderm.

Cytotrophoblast

Blastocele

Amniotic Cavity

Endoderm

Ectoderm

Syncytiotrophoblast

Nucleus

DEVELOPMENT / Embryonic Development

DEVELOPMENTAL CHANGES

In humans, the developing organism is called an *embryo* from the second week after fertilization (when the three primary germ layers form) through the eighth week (when the organism develops a human shape). The following is a short outline of some of the changes that occur during the embryonic stage of development.

2nd Week A bilaminar (double-layered) embryonic disc forms, consisting of ectoderm and endoderm. Extraembryonic mesoderm forms. Two fluid-filled cavities form: the amniotic cavity and the extraembryonic coelom. The yolk sac forms. The chorion, which consists of the cytotrophoblast and syncytiotrophoblast, forms, and surrounds the other developing structures.

3rd Week A trilaminar (triple-layered) embryonic disc forms, consisting of ectoderm, endoderm, and mesoderm. The heart develops and begins to beat. A primitive nervous system forms (neural folds and notochord). A primitive digestive tract forms.

4th Week A three-vesicle brain develops. Upper and lower limb buds appear. The maxillary and mandibular processes appear. The eyes, ears, and trachea begin to develop.

5th Week A five-vesicle brain develops. Hand plates and paddle-shaped lower limbs develop. A distinct head and tail develop. The face begins to develop. Internal organs continue to develop.

6th Week The head and brain enlarge. The hand plates develop digital rays and foot plates develop. Sensory organs develop and a pigmented eye appears. The gonads are prominent, but undifferentiated.

7th Week Eyelids begin to form and the external ears develop. The legs and toe rays develop. The heart becomes partitioned, forming a four-chambered heart. The primitive digestive tract divides, forming the rectum, urinary bladder, and primitive reproductive organs.

8th Week By the eighth week, most of the body organs are formed. The gonads are differentiated into testes or ovaries; but the external genitals remain undifferentiated. The nose, eyes, and auditory canals develop. The feet and hands develop. The embryonic stage ends at the end of the 8th week. At this time, the embryo is about 1 inch (30 mm) long.

MAJOR EVENTS

Three major events occur during the embryonic period of development.

Primary Germ Layers The first major event of the embryonic period is the formation of three primary germ layers. They are the embryonic tissues from which all tissues and organs of the body will ultimately develop. Early in the embryonic period the inner cell mass of the blastocyts differentiates into ectoderm, endoderm, and mesoderm.

Embryonic Membranes The second major event of the embryonic period is the formation of embryonic (extraembryonic) membranes. The four embryonic membranes are the yolk sac, amnion, chorion, and allantois.

Placenta The third major event of the embryonic period is the development of the placenta. The placenta is formed by the 3rd month of pregnancy. It allows for the exchange of materials between the blood of the mother and the fetus.

EMBRYONIC DEVELOPMENT

The 2nd week through the end of the 8th week

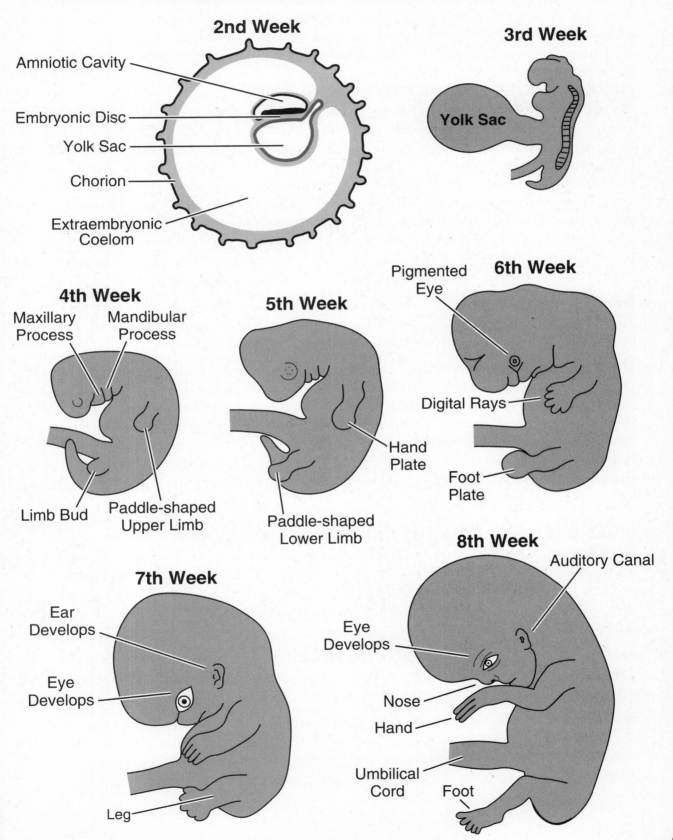

2nd Week

Amniotic Cavity

Embryonic Disc

Yolk Sac

Chorion

Extraembryonic Coelom

3rd Week

Yolk Sac

4th Week

Maxillary Process

Mandibular Process

Limb Bud

Paddle-shaped Upper Limb

5th Week

Hand Plate

Paddle-shaped Lower Limb

6th Week

Pigmented Eye

Digital Rays

Foot Plate

7th Week

Ear Develops

Eye Develops

Leg

8th Week

Auditory Canal

Eye Develops

Nose

Hand

Umbilical Cord

Foot

DEVELOPMENT / Primary Germ Layers

Primary Germ Layers The first major event of the embryonic stage of development is the formation of the three primary germ layers: ectoderm, endoderm, and mesoderm. These are the embryonic tissues from which all tissues and organs of the body will develop.

Gastrulation The cell migrations that establish the primary germ layers are called gastrulation.

DEVELOPMENT DURING THE SECOND WEEK

Day 7 By day 7, the *blastocyst* has implanted in the lining of the uterus (endometrium). The *trophoblast* (the outer covering of cells of the blastocyst) differentiates into two types of tissues in the region of contact between the blastocyst and endometrium: an outer *syncytiotrophoblast* and an inner *cytotrophoblast*.

The *inner cell mass* of the blastocyst differentiates into two primary germ layers: *ectoderm* and *endoderm*. The top layer of cells of the inner cell mass proliferates, forming a ball of cells with a fluid-filled space (the amniotic cavity). The cells closest to the cytotrophoblast differentiate into the amnion (an embryonic membrane); the cells closest to the blastocoele differentiate into *ectoderm*. The bottom layer of cells of the inner cell mass differentiate into *endoderm*. The layers of endoderm and ectoderm form a bilaminar (double-layered) *embryonic disc*.

Day 12 By day 12, the endoderm cells have proliferated, forming the *yolk sac* (another embryonic membrane). Cells of the mesoderm begin to appear between the yolk sac and the cytotrophoblast; this type of mesoderm is called *extraembryonic mesoderm*.

Day 14 About day 14, the cells of the embryonic disc differentiate into three distinct layers: the upper ectoderm, the middle mesoderm, and the lower endoderm. The *embryonic disc* is now trilaminar (triple-layered). These three layers of primary germ cells make up the *embryo* at its earliest stage of development. The *extraembryonic mesoderm* proliferates and forms a layer inside the cytotrophoblast; this forms a new cavity called the *extraembryonic coelom*, which surrounds the embryonic disc, amniotic cavity, and yolk sac. The extraembryonic mesoderm also forms a *body stalk* between the embryo and the cytotrophoblast, which will become the *umbilical cord*.

TISSUES DERIVED FROM THE PRIMARY GERM LAYERS

Ectoderm All nervous tissue; epidermis of the skin; hair follicles; arrector pili muscles, nails, and epithelium of skin glands (sebaceous and sudoriferous); lens, cornea, and internal eye muscles; internal and external ear; neuroepithelium of sense organs; epithelium of the oral cavity, nasal cavity, paranasal sinuses, salivary glands, anal canal, pineal gland, pituitary gland, and adrenal medulla.

Endoderm Epithelium of the gastrointestinal tract, respiratory tract, urinary bladder, thyroid gland, parathyroid gland, thymus gland, male prostate and bulbourethral glands, vestibule (of the vulva), vagina, and vestibular glands (of the vagina).

Mesoderm All skeletal, most smooth, and all cardiac muscle; cartilage, bone, and other connective tissues; blood, bone marrow, and lymphoid tissue; endothelium of blood vessels and lymphatics; dermis of skin; fibrous tunic and vascular tunic of eye; middle ear; joint cavities; epithelium of kidneys, adrenal cortex, gonads, and genital ducts.

PRIMARY GERM LAYERS

Simplified Illustration
(individual cells not shown)

Day 7

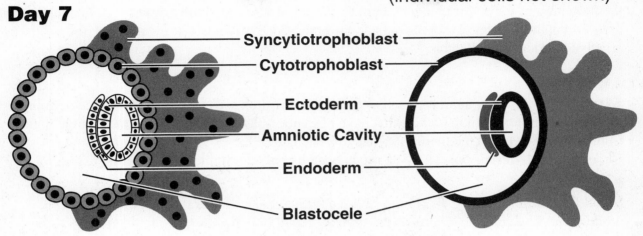

- Syncytiotrophoblast
- Cytotrophoblast
- Ectoderm
- Amniotic Cavity
- Endoderm
- Blastocele

Day 12

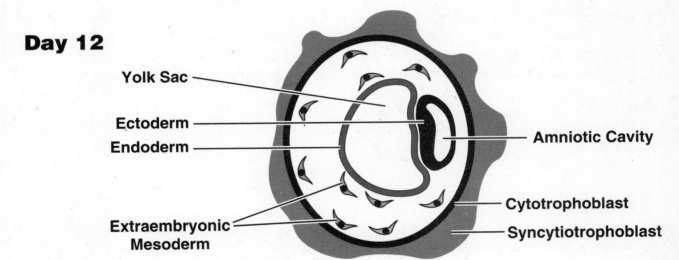

- Yolk Sac
- Ectoderm
- Endoderm
- Extraembryonic Mesoderm
- Amniotic Cavity
- Cytotrophoblast
- Syncytiotrophoblast

Day 14 (2 Weeks)

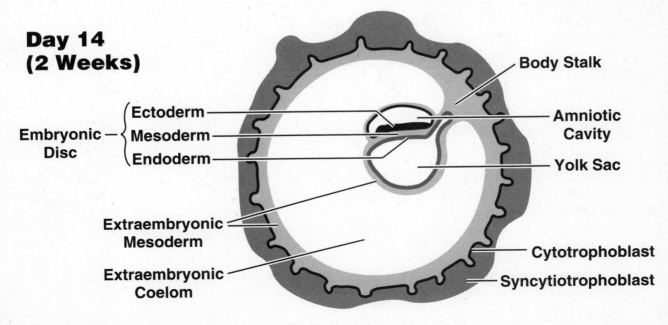

- Embryonic Disc
  - Ectoderm
  - Mesoderm
  - Endoderm
- Extraembryonic Mesoderm
- Extraembryonic Coelom
- Body Stalk
- Amniotic Cavity
- Yolk Sac
- Cytotrophoblast
- Syncytiotrophoblast

DEVELOPMENT / Embryonic Membranes

Embryonic Membranes   The second major event that occurs during embryonic development is the formation of the embryonic membranes. They are also called the extraembryonic membranes (*extra* = outside), because they lie outside the embryo.   There are four membranes: the yolk sac, amnion, chorion, and allantois.

YOLK SAC
Structure   In many animals (such as chickens), the yolk sac is the primary source of nourishment for the embryo. In mammals that have placentas (placental mammals), most of the nourishment is provided by the mother, so the yolk sac is small.
Endoderm and *Mesoderm*   The yolk sac is lined by endoderm; the outer layer is mesoderm.

Functions
Blood Formation   During embryonic and fetal life, there are several centers for blood cell production. The yolk sac, liver, spleen, thymus gland, lymph nodes, and bone marrow all participate at various times in the production of red blood cells and white blood cells.
Primordial Germ Cells   Early in embryonic development, some of the endoderm cells lining the yolk sac differentiate into primordial germ cells. These cells migrate to the developing testes in males and ovaries in females, where they become spermatogonia and oogonia, respectively.
Umbilical Cord   The yolk sac becomes a nonfunctional part of the umbilical cord.

AMNION
Structure   The amnion is a thin, protective membrane that forms by the 8th day after fertilization. Initially, it overlies the embryonic disc. The amnion eventually surrounds the embryo, creating a fluid-filled cavity called the *amniotic cavity*.
Ectoderm and *Mesoderm*   The amnion is lined by ectoderm; the outer layer is mesoderm.

Functions
Amniotic fluid serves as a shock absorber for the fetus, helps regulate fetal body temperature, and prevents adhesions (attachments) between the skin of the fetus and surrounding tissues.
Amniocentesis   Embryonic cells are sloughed off into the amniotic fluid and can be examined by a procedure called amniocentesis.
"Bag of Waters"   The amnion usually ruptures just before birth; together with its fluid, it is often referred to as the "bag of waters."

CHORION
Structure   The chorion is the outermost embryonic membrane. It surrounds the amnion and eventually fuses with it.
Trophoblast and *Mesoderm*   The chorion is lined with mesoderm; the outer layer is trophoblast.

Function
Placenta (Embryonic Portion)   The chorion forms the embryonic portion of the placenta.

ALLANTOIS
Structure   The allantois is an outpocketing of the yolk sac, so it is lined by endoderm.

Function   In animals that do not have a placenta, the allantois serves as a storage place for metabolic wastes. In humans, it serves as an early site for blood formation and eventually becomes part of the umbilical cord.

EMBRYONIC MEMBRANES

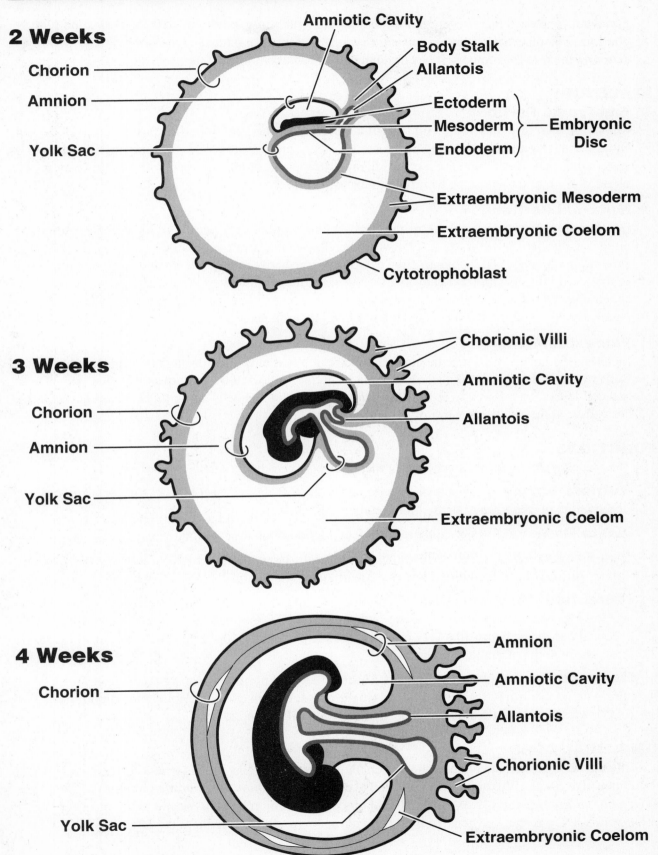

2 Weeks

Amniotic Cavity

Chorion

Amnion

Yolk Sac

Body Stalk

Allantois

Ectoderm

Mesoderm

Endoderm

Embryonic Disc

Extraembryonic Mesoderm

Extraembryonic Coelom

Cytotrophoblast

3 Weeks

Chorion

Amnion

Yolk Sac

Chorionic Villi

Amniotic Cavity

Allantois

Extraembryonic Coelom

4 Weeks

Chorion

Yolk Sac

Amnion

Amniotic Cavity

Allantois

Chorionic Villi

Extraembryonic Coelom

DEVELOPMENT / Placenta

Placenta   The third major event that occurs during embryonic development is the formation of the placenta. The placenta consists of the *chorion* of the embryo and the *decidua basalis* (a portion of the endometrium) of the mother. It has the shape of a flat cake.

STRUCTURE
Embryonic Portion
Chorionic Villi The chorionic villi (singular: chorionic villus) are fingerlike projections of the chorion that extend into the lining of the uterus. Thus, embryonic tissues become interwoven with maternal tissues. Fetal blood vessels fill the internal spaces of the chorionic villi. In this way fetal blood is brought into close proximity with maternal blood.

Maternal Portion
Decidua Basalis (of the Endometrium) The decidua basalis is the portion of the endometrium that directly underlies the embryo. It is between the chorion and stratum basalis.
Intervillous Spaces   The regions of the decidua basilis between the villi are dissolved by enzymes, so that each villus is surrounded by sinuses (spaces) filled with maternal blood; these spaces are called intervillous spaces (*inter* = between). The two blood supplies, fetal and maternal, are separated only by a thin membrane called the placental membrane.

Placental Membrane
Materials exchanged between the maternal and fetal blood must pass through the cells that line the walls of the villi and the endothelial cells that form the walls of the capillaries inside the villi. These two cell layers are referred to as the placental membrane. (The cells lining the walls of the villi are derived from the cytotrophoblast of the embryo).

FUNCTIONS
The placenta allows for the exchange of materials between the blood of the mother and the fetus.

Nutrient Supply   Nutrients diffuse into fetal blood from maternal blood. Nutrients are also stored in the placenta, and released into fetal circulation as required.

Waste Removal Wastes diffuse from fetal blood into maternal blood.

Gas Exchange   Oxygen diffuses into fetal blood from maternal blood; simultaneously, carbon dioxide diffuses from fetal blood into maternal blood.

Protection   The placenta serves as a protective barrier, since most microorganisms cannot cross it. However, certain viruses, such as those that cause AIDS, German measles, chickenpox, measles, encephalitis, and poliomyelitis may pass through the placenta. Most drugs, including alcohol, pass freely through the placenta.

Hormone Production   The placenta secretes several hormones during pregnancy: human chorionic gonadotropin (hCG); estrogen; progesterone; human chorionic somatomammotropin (hCS), which is also called human placental lactogen (hPL); and relaxin.

UMBILICAL CORD
The umbilical cord that connects the placenta to the fetus contains blood vessels surrounded by connective tissue (Wharton's jelly), and is covered by the *amniotic membrane* (amnion). Two *umbilical arteries* carry deoxygenated fetal blood containing metabolic wastes to the placenta; one *umbilical vein* carries oxygenated blood and nutrients from the placenta to the fetus.

PLACENTA AND DECIDUA

Pregnant Uterus

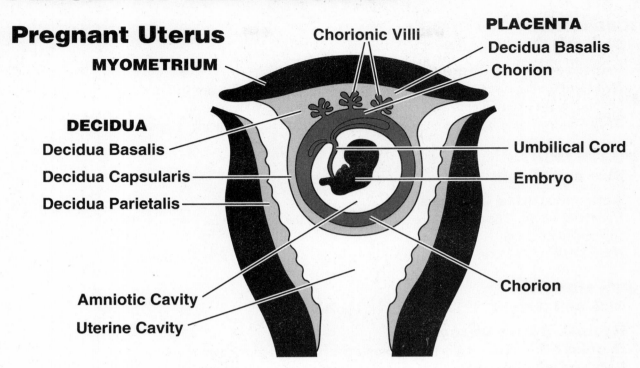

Chorionic Villi

PLACENTA
Decidua Basalis
Chorion

MYOMETRIUM

DECIDUA
Decidua Basalis
Decidua Capsularis
Decidua Parietalis

Umbilical Cord
Embryo

Chorion

Amniotic Cavity
Uterine Cavity

Placenta (detail)
Umbilical arteries not shown.

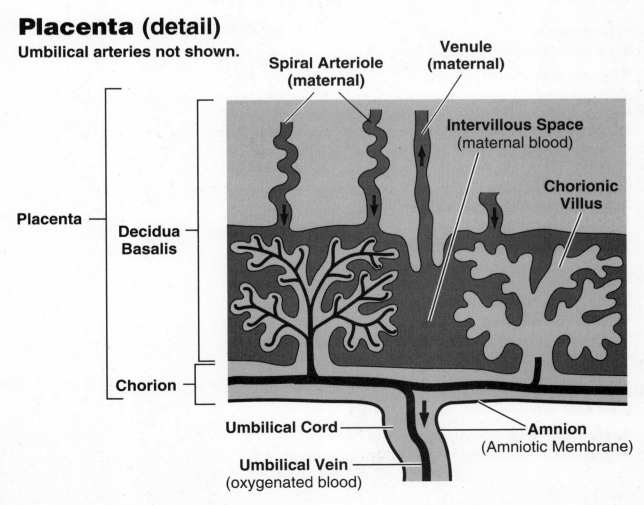

Spiral Arteriole
(maternal)

Venule
(maternal)

Intervillous Space
(maternal blood)

Chorionic
Villus

Placenta

Decidua
Basalis

Chorion

Umbilical Cord

Amnion
(Amniotic Membrane)

Umbilical Vein
(oxygenated blood)

DEVELOPMENT / Fetal Development

THIRD MONTH
Size and Weight 3 inches; 1 ounce.

Representative Changes
Head and Limbs Eyes are almost fully developed, but the eyelids are still fused; the nose develops the bridge; the external ears are present. The limbs are fully formed.
Body Systems Heartbeat can be detected; urine starts to form; bone development continues.

FOURTH MONTH
Size and Weight 7 inches; 4 ounces.

Representative Changes
Head and Limbs The head is large in proportion to the body; the face takes on human features; hair appears on the head.
Body Systems The skin is bright pink; many bones are ossified; joints begin to form.

FIFTH MONTH
Size and Weight 12 inches (1 foot); 1 pound.

Representative Changes
Head and Limbs The head is less disproportionate. Fetal movement is commonly felt.
Body Systems Lanugo (fine hair) covers the body; skin is still bright pink; brown fat forms.

SIXTH MONTH
Size and Weight 14 inches; 1 1/2 pounds.

Representative Changes
Head and Limbs The head becomes even less disproportionate to the rest of the body. Eyelids separate and eyelashes form.
Body Systems Alveolar cells in the lungs begin to produce surfactant; skin is wrinkled and pink.

SEVENTH MONTH
Size and Weight 17 inches; 3 pounds.

Representative Changes
Head and Limbs The head and body are proportionate. Fetus assumes an upside-down position.
Body Systems The skin is wrinkled and pink.

EIGHTH MONTH
Size and Weight 18 inches; 5 pounds.

Representative Changes
Body Systems Testes descend in males; skin is less wrinkled; bones of the head are soft; subcutaneous fat is deposited.

NINTH MONTH
Size and Weight 20 inches; 7 1/2 pounds.

Representative Changes
Body Systems Lanugo (fine hair) is shed; nails extend to the tips of fingers; fat accumulates.

FETAL STAGE

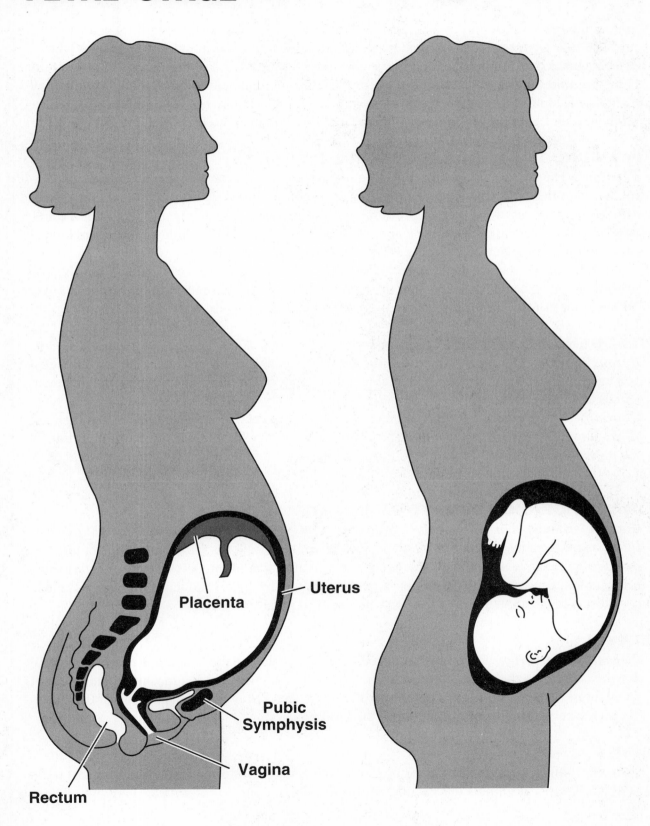

Placenta

Uterus

Pubic
Symphysis

Vagina

Rectum

DEVELOPMENT / Hormones of Pregnancy

During the first two months of pregnancy, the uterine lining is maintained by estrogen and progesterone secreted by the corpus luteum. During the last seven months of pregnancy, the placenta takes over the production of estrogen and progesterone. The high levels of progesterone in the presence of estrogen inhibit the secretion of GnRH (gonadotropin-releasing hormone) by the hypothalamus; consequently, gonadotropins (FSH and LH) are not released by the anterior pituitary gland, no follicles develop in the ovaries, and there are no menstrual cycles.

HUMAN CHORIONIC GONADOTROPIN (hCG)

Chorion   The chorion (trophoblast in the embryo) begins to secrete human chorionic gonadotropin (hCG) by the 8th day after fertilization. It mimics LH, stimulating the production of estrogen and progesterone by the corpus luteum. High levels of estrogen and progesterone are necessary for the continued attachment of the embryo and fetus to the lining of the uterus. Peak secretion of hCG occurs at about the 9th week of pregnancy.

During the 4th month, the hCG level decreases sharply, then levels off until childbirth. This is because the placenta has taken over the function of secreting estrogen and progesterone, so the the secretions of the corpus luteum are no longer essential.

ESTROGEN AND PROGESTERONE

Corpus Luteum   During the first three months of pregnancy, the corpus luteum secretes estrogen and progesterone, hormones that maintain the lining of the uterus and prepare the mammary glands to secrete milk.

Chorion   During embryonic development, the chorion secretes small quantities of estrogen and progesterone. During fetal development (from the 3rd to the 9th month), the chorion portion of the placenta supplies the estrogen and progesterone needed to maintain the pregnancy and develop the mammary glands for lactation.

HUMAN CHORIONIC SOMATOMAMMOTROPIN (hCS)

Chorion   *Human chorionic somatomammotropin (hCS)*, also called *human placental lactogen (hPL)*, is released by the chorion portion of the placenta. It reaches maximum levels in the 4th month of pregnancy and remains relatively constant after that. It prepares the mammary glands for lactation, causes growth (maintains a positive protein balance), maintains high plasma glucose levels to meet the needs of the fetus, and mobilizes fat for energy.

RELAXIN

Placenta and Ovaries   Relaxin is produced by the placenta and the ovaries. Near the time of delivery, it relaxes the pubic symphysis (the cartilagenous joint between the anterior surfaces of the hipbones) and the ligaments of the sacroiliac and sacrococcygeal joints. It also softens and dilates the cervix, facilitating parturition (the birth process).

INHIBIN

Ovaries   Inhibin, which is produced by the ovaries (and the testes in the male), is present in the placenta at term. It inhibits the secretion of follicle-stimulating hormone (FSH).

HORMONAL CHANGES

Hormonal Changes During Pregnancy

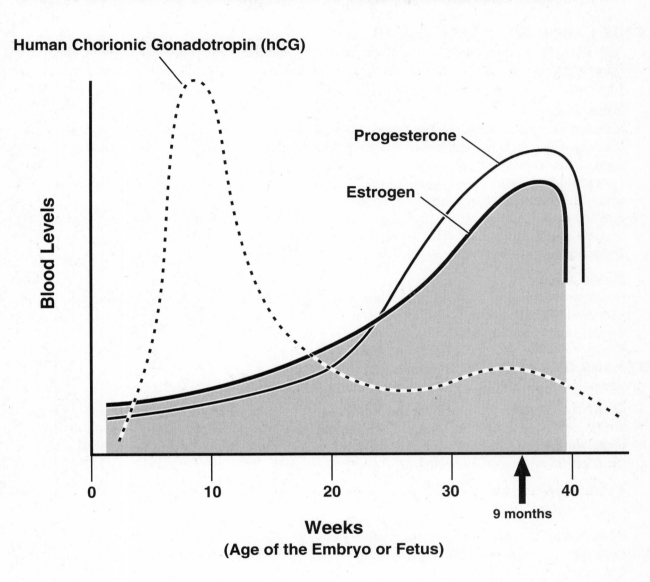

Human Chorionic Gonadotropin (hCG)

Progesterone

Estrogen

Blood Levels

0   10   20   30   40

9 months

Weeks
(Age of the Embryo or Fetus)

DEVELOPMENT / Birth

Gestation   Gestation is the period of development from the time of fertilization until birth. In humans, the gestation period is about 266 days.

Labor   The process of giving birth. The fetus is expelled from the uterus into the vagina and then outside the body. Labor is also called *childbirth*, *parturition*, *delivery*, *confinement*, and *travail*.

TRUE LABOR AND FALSE LABOR

Just before birth, the muscles of the uterus contract rhythmically and forcefully. Uterine contractions occur in waves, quite similar to peristaltic waves, that start at the top of the uterus and move downward. These waves expel the fetus.

True Labor

Regular Intervals and Increasing Intensity of Contractions   True labor begins when uterine contractions occur at regular intervals, usually producing pain. As the intervals between contractions shorten, the contractions intensify.

Localization of Pain   Another sign of true labor in some females is localization of pain in the back, which is intensified by walking.

The "Show"   The "show" is a discharge of a blood-containing mucus that accumulates in the cervical canal during labor. This is another sign of true labor.

Dilation of the Cervix   Another reliable indication of true labor is the dilation of the cervix.

False Labor

Irregular Intervals of Pain   In false labor, pain is felt in the abdomen at irregular intervals. The pain does not intensify and is not altered significantly by walking. There is no "show" and no cervical dilation.

STAGES OF LABOR

Labor can be divided into three stages: dilation; expulsion; and the placental stage.

Dilation Stage   The time from the onset of labor to the complete dilation of the cervix is called the dilation stage. During this stage, there are regular contractions of the uterus, usually a rupturing of the amniotic sac ("bag of waters"), and complete dilation (10 cm) of the cervix. If the amniotic sac does not rupture spontaneously, it is done deliberately.

Expulsion Stage   The time from complete cervical dilation to delivery of the baby is called the expulsion stage.

Placental Stage   The time after delivery until the placenta or "afterbirth" is expelled by powerful uterine contractions is called the placental state. These contractions also constrict blood vessels that were torn during delivery, thus reducing the chance of hemorrhage (bleeding).

HORMONAL CONTROL

Several hormones are involved in labor.

Estrogen and Progesterone   At the end of gestation, the high progesterone level, which inhibits uterine contractions, falls. The estrogen level in the maternal blood is now sufficient to overcome the inhibiting effects of progesterone, and labor begins.

Cortisol   Cortisol, released by the fetus, also blocks the inhibiting effects of progesterone.

Oxytocin   Oxytocin from the posterior pituitary gland stimulates uterine contractions.

Relaxin   Relaxin dilates the uterine cervix and relaxes the pubic symphysis.

Prostaglandins   Prostaglandins may also play a role in labor.

STAGES OF LABOR

Dilation Stage

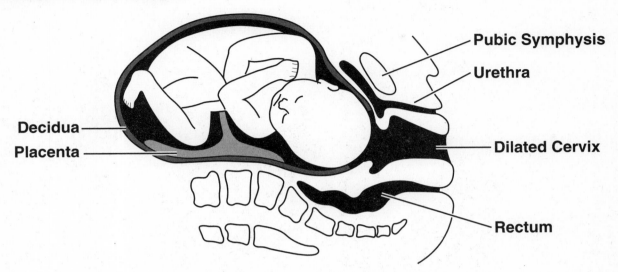

Expulsion Stage

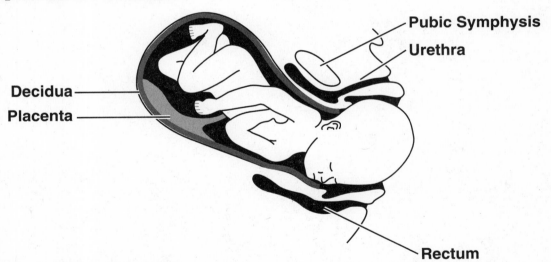

Placental Stage

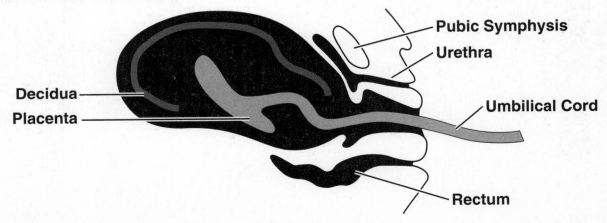

Part II : Self-Testing Exercises

Unlabeled illustrations from Part I

FERTILIZATION

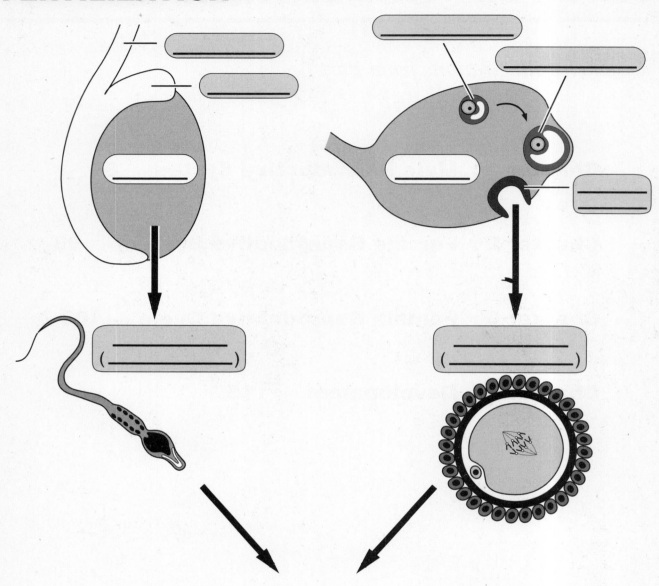

Fertilization

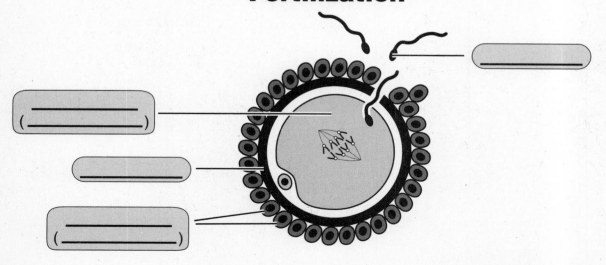

TESTES

Anatomy

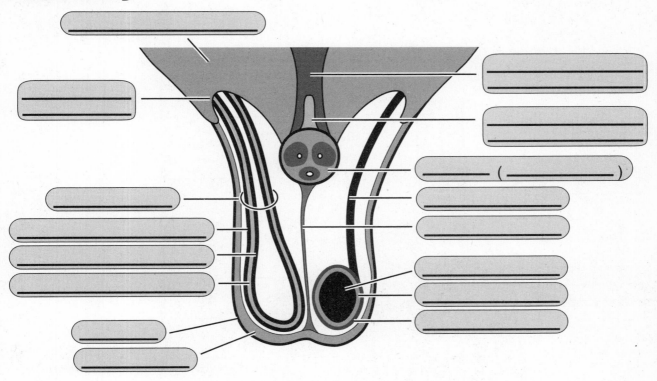

Location

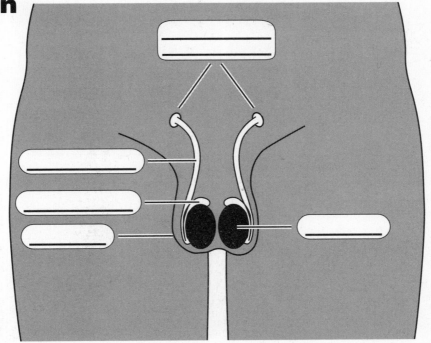

TESTES : Tubules
Sagittal section of a testis

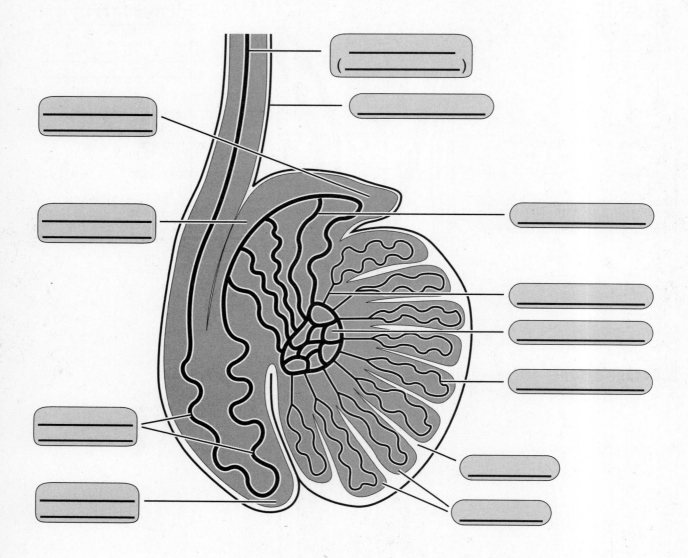

SEMINIFEROUS TUBULES

An Area Of Testis (cross–section)

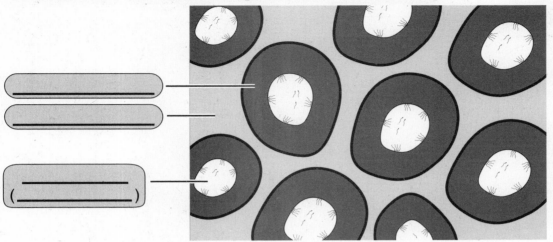

Wall of Tubule (detail)

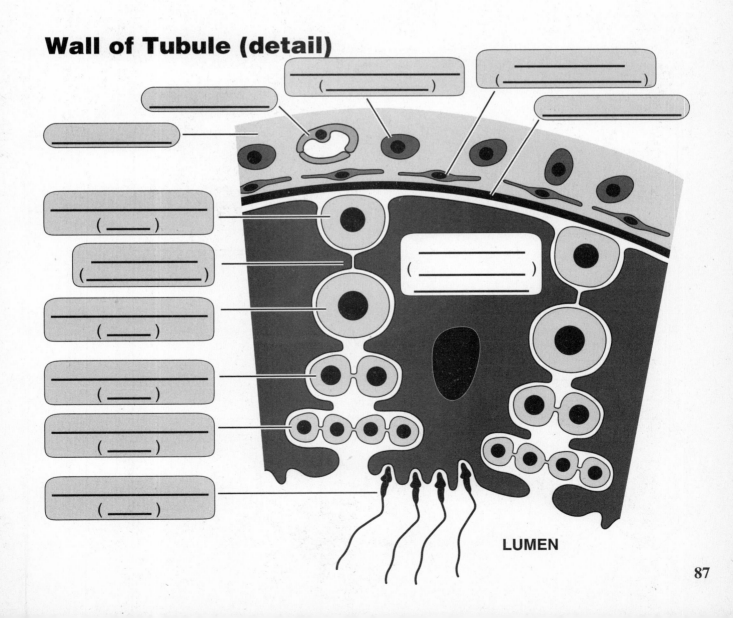

LUMEN

GAMETOGENESIS

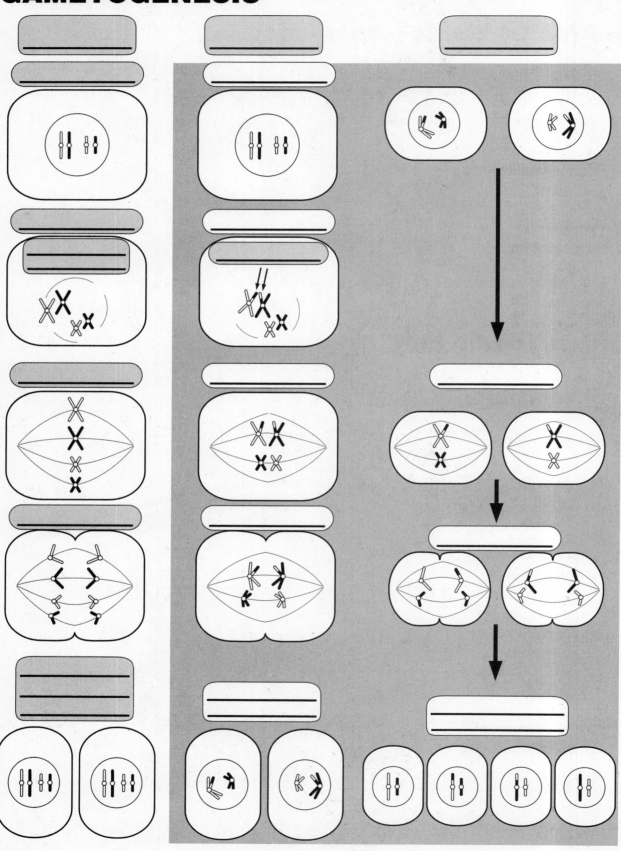

SPERMATOGENESIS

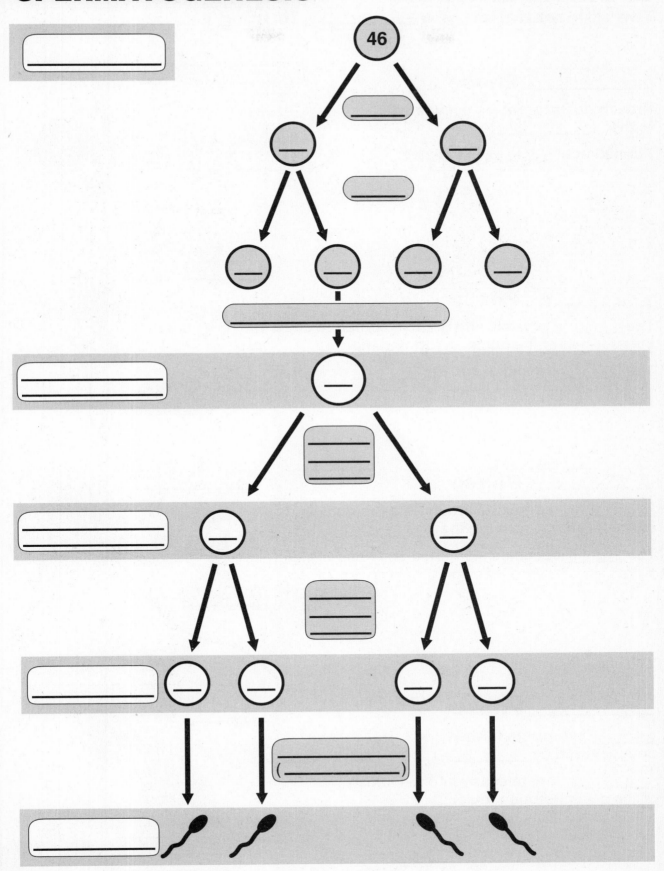

SPERMIOGENESIS

The differentiation of a _____ , forming a _____ .

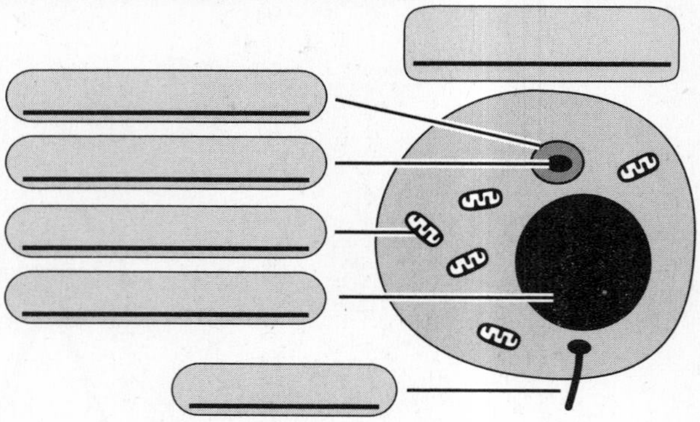

_____ Phase

Proacrosomal granules accumulate in the _____.

Formation of _____ is initiated.

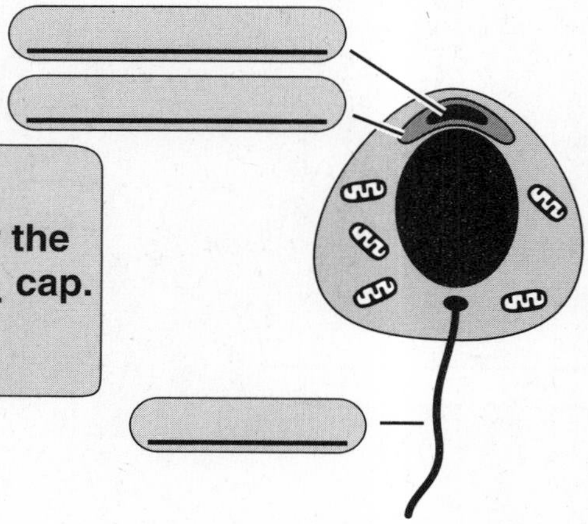

_____ Phase

The _____ vesicle and granule spread to cover the anterior half of the nucleus, forming the _____ cap.

The _____ elongates and the _____ develops.

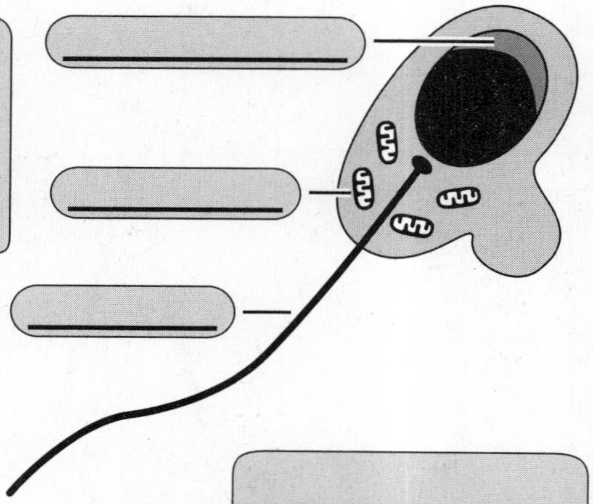

_____ Phase

_____ aggregate around the proximal end of the flagellum, forming the _____ .

The _____ becomes elongated and condensed.

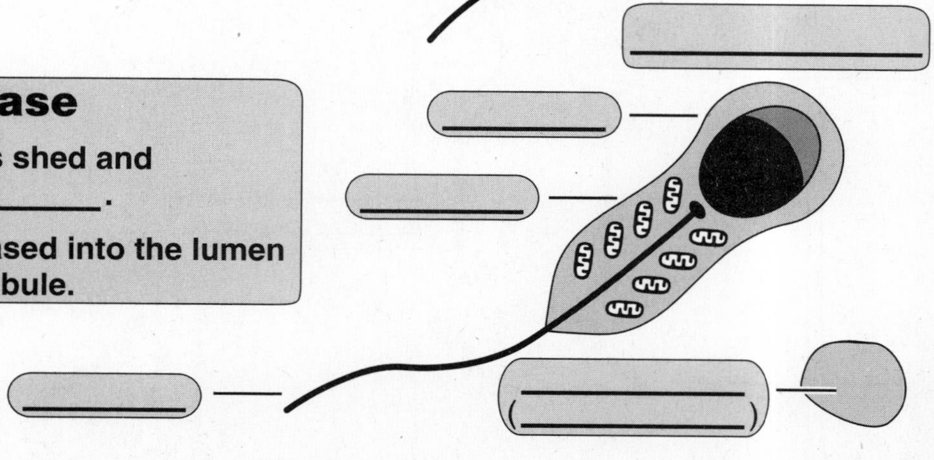

_____ Phase

_____ cytoplasm is shed and phagocytized by _____.

_____ are released into the lumen of the seminiferous tubule.

90

HUMAN SPERMATOZOON

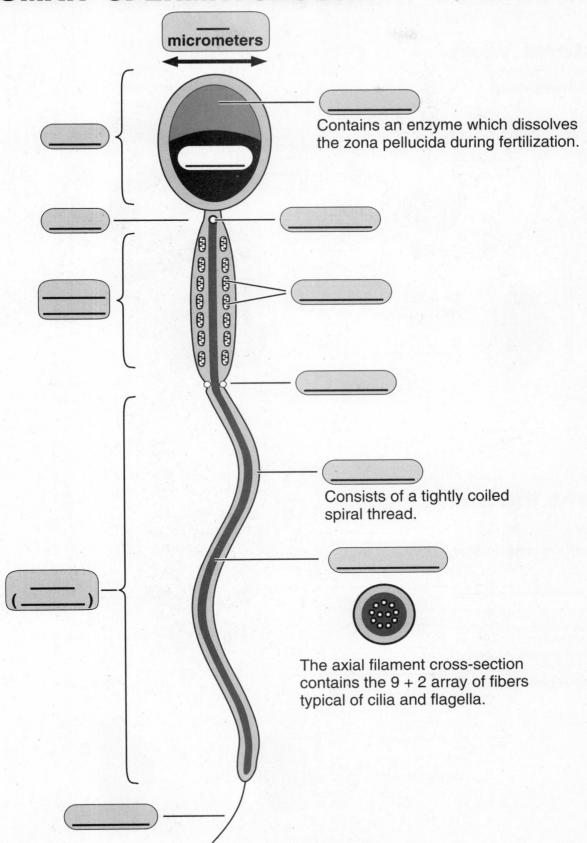

micrometers

Contains an enzyme which dissolves the zona pellucida during fertilization.

Consists of a tightly coiled spiral thread.

The axial filament cross-section contains the 9 + 2 array of fibers typical of cilia and flagella.

DUCTS AND GLANDS

Lateral View

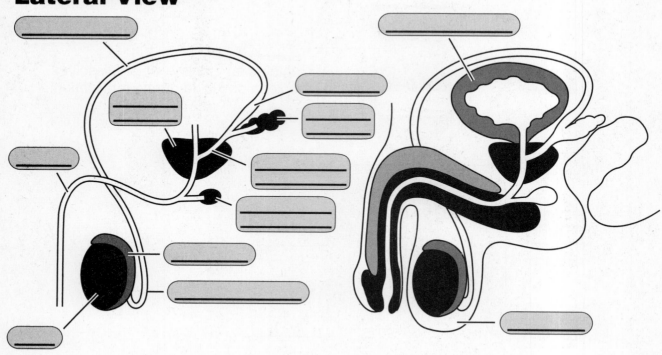

Front View

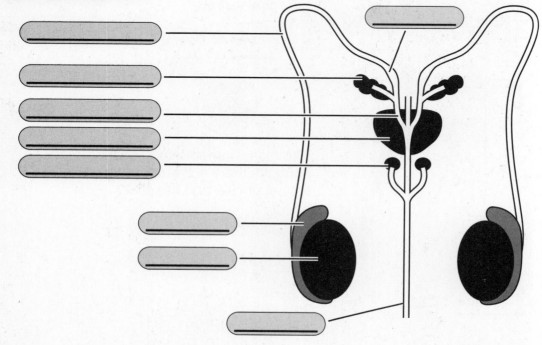

MALE REPRODUCTIVE ORGANS
Sagittal Section

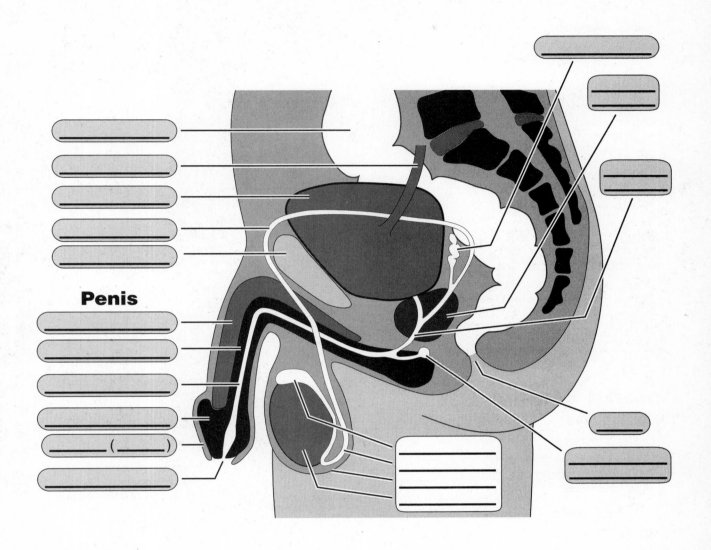

Penis

PENIS

Cross Section

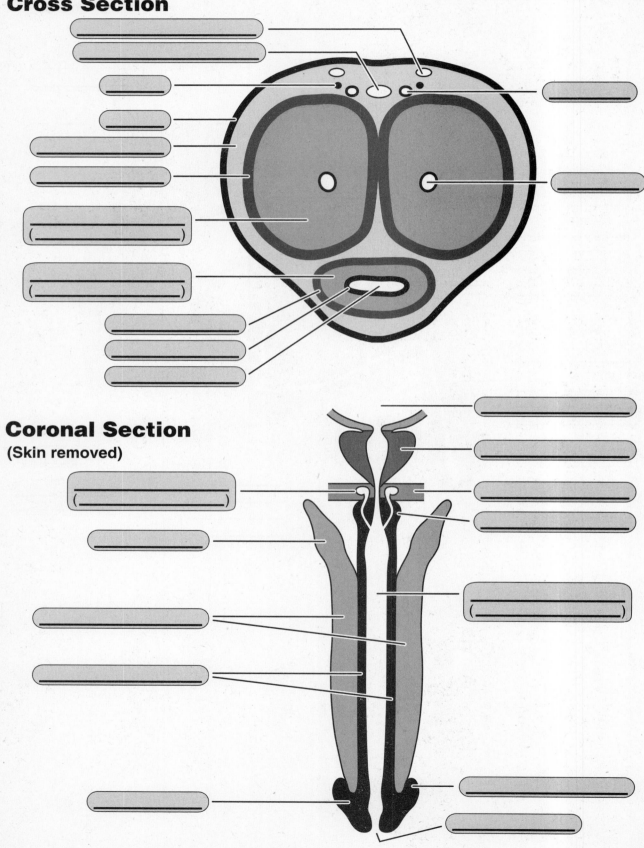

Coronal Section

(Skin removed)

ERECTION

Reflex Pathway

_____ tissue fills with blood.

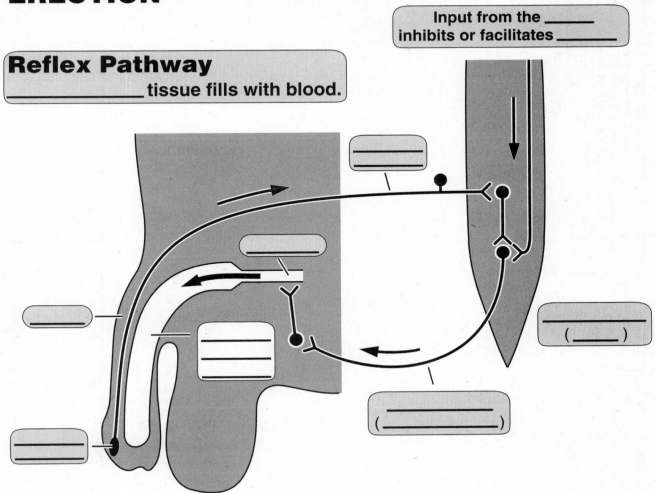

_____ Dilate
(_____ constrict passively)

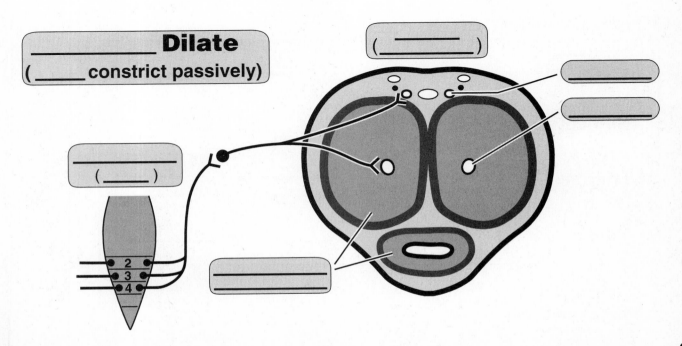

SEMEN

Characteristics

Volume	___ to ___ ml per ejaculation
Color	_____ appearance (due to prostatic secretion)
Sperm Count	___ to ____ million sperm per ml
Motility	at least ___% active (show good forward motility)
pH	slightly_____ (ranges between 7.20 and 7.60)
Specific Gravity	_____ (denser than water)
Morphology	at least ___% normal (fewer than 20% abnormal forms)

Other Components

Antibiotics	_____
Nutrients	_____
Enzymes	_____, _____, _____, and _____
Buffers	_____ and _____

MALE REPRODUCTIVE HORMONES

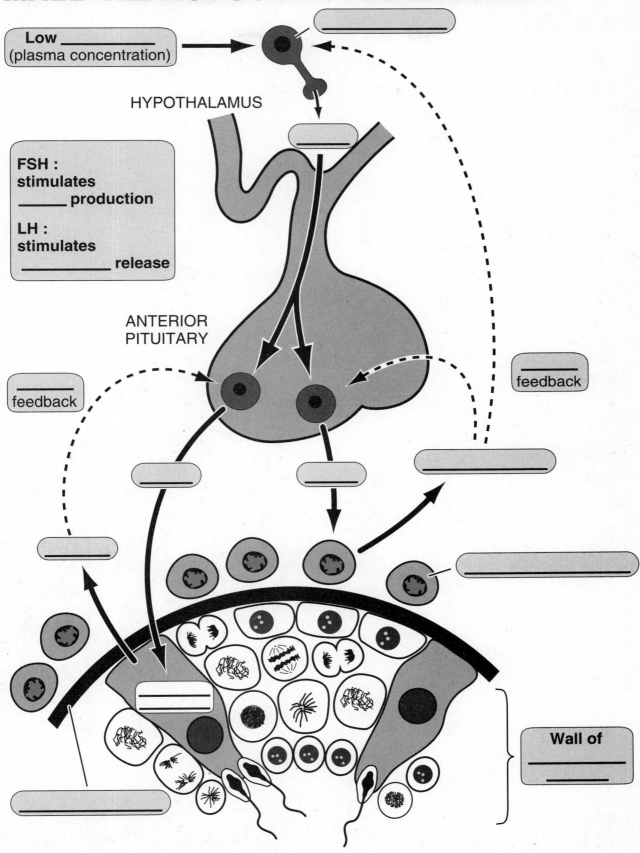

Low _____
(plasma concentration)

HYPOTHALAMUS

FSH :
stimulates
_____ production

LH :
stimulates
_____ release

ANTERIOR
PITUITARY

_____
feedback

_____
feedback

Wall of

_____
_____

FEMALE REPRODUCTIVE ORGANS
Front View

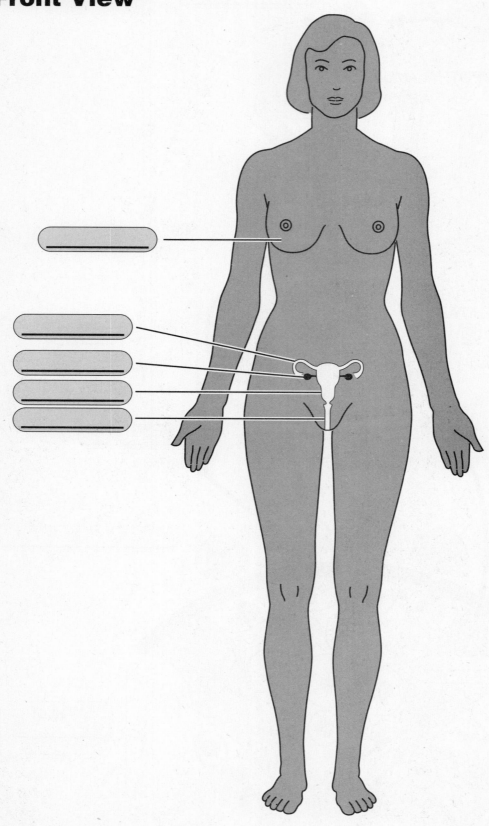

OVARY

Ovarian Cycle

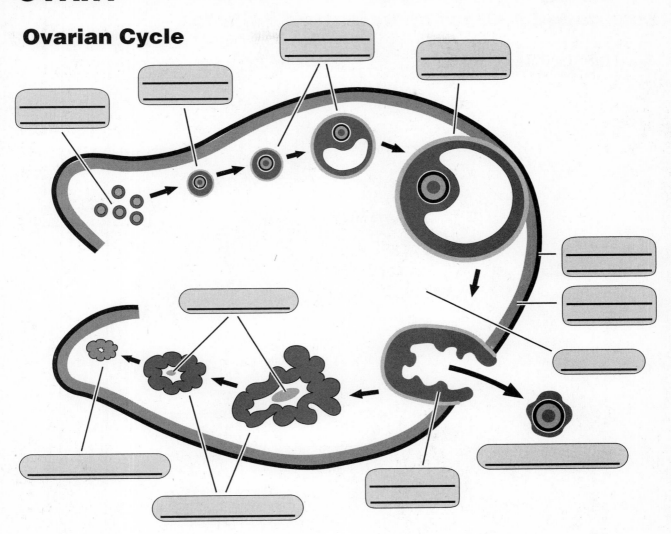

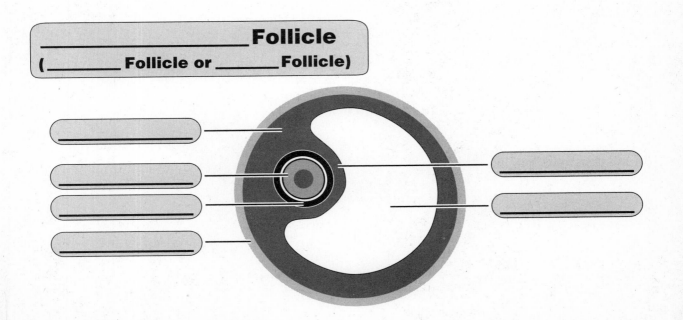

_____**Follicle**
(_____ **Follicle or** _____ **Follicle)**

VESICULAR OVARIAN FOLLICLE
also called a Graafian or Mature Follicle

A mature follicle contains a _____ oocyte in _____ of meiosis II.

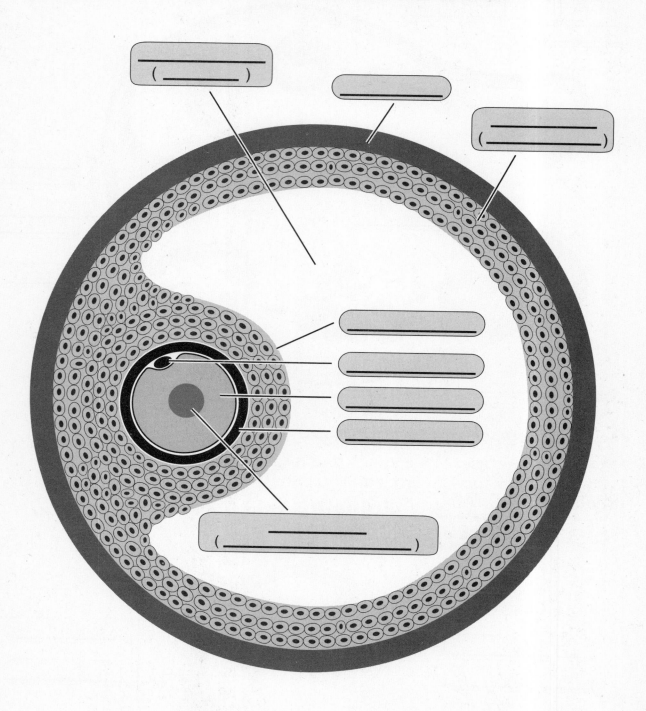

(   )

(   )

(   )

MATURE OVUM (EGG)

At the time of _____ , a mature follicle ruptures, propelling a
_____ from an ovary into a _____ .

Some of the _____ (follicular) cells remain attached to the oocyte,
forming a structure called the _____ .

```
[ _____ ]
( _____ )

[ _____ ]

[ _____ ]

[ _____
( _____ ) ]
```

Sperm

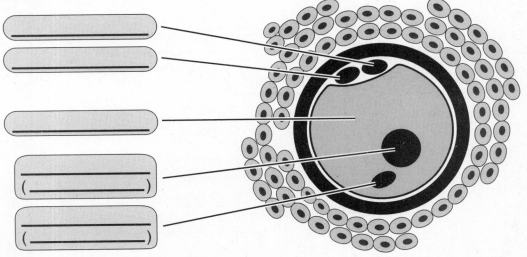

After _____ , the secondary oocyte completes _____ ,
forming a small daughter cell (the _____) and
a large daughter cell (the _____).

The haploid nuclei of the sperm and the ovum are called _____ .
The pronuclei fuse to form the diploid nucleus (_____)
of the zygote.

```
[ _____ ]
[ _____ ]

[ _____ ]

[ _____
( _____ ) ]

[ _____
( _____ ) ]
```

OOGENESIS
Production of an Ovum by Meiosis

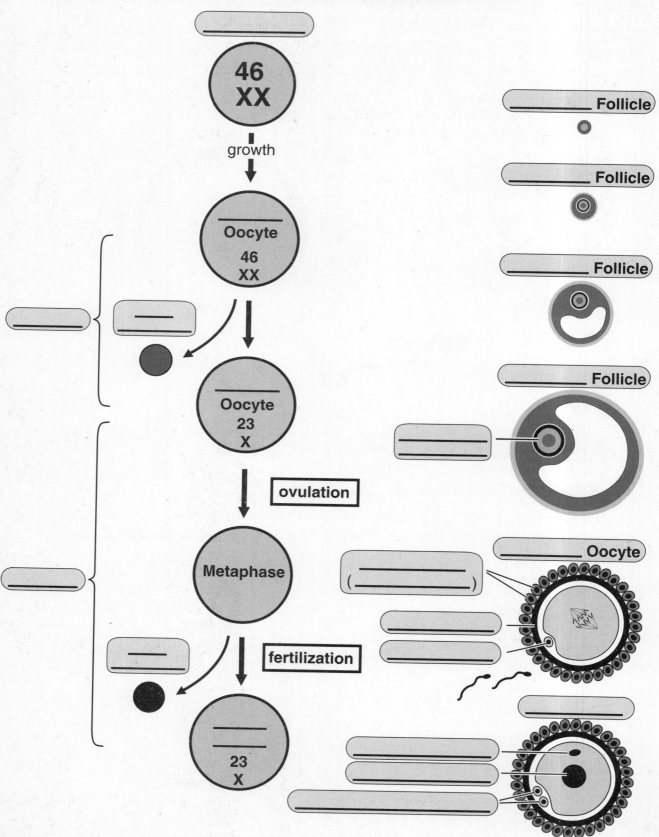

46
XX

growth

Oocyte
46
XX

Oocyte
23
X

ovulation

Metaphase

fertilization

23
X

Follicle

Follicle

Follicle

Follicle

Oocyte

FEMALE REPRODUCTIVE ORGANS
Sagittal Section

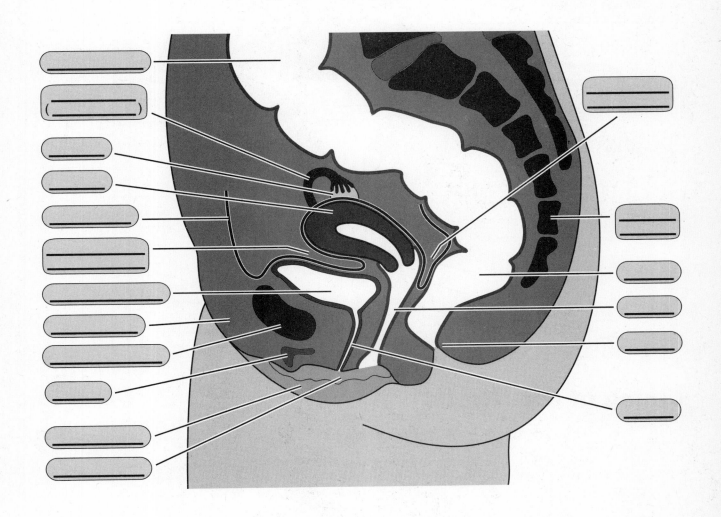

UTERUS

Uterus and Associated Structures

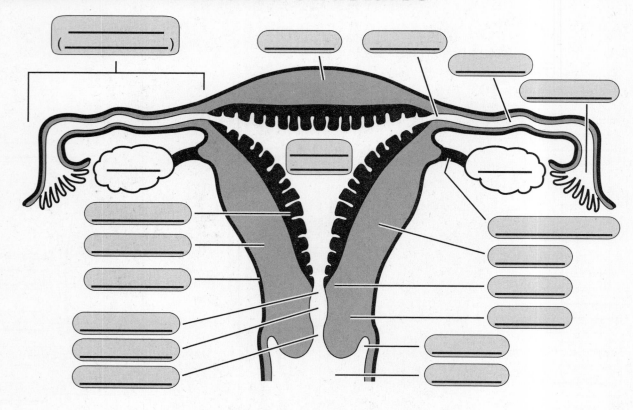

Lining of the Uterus

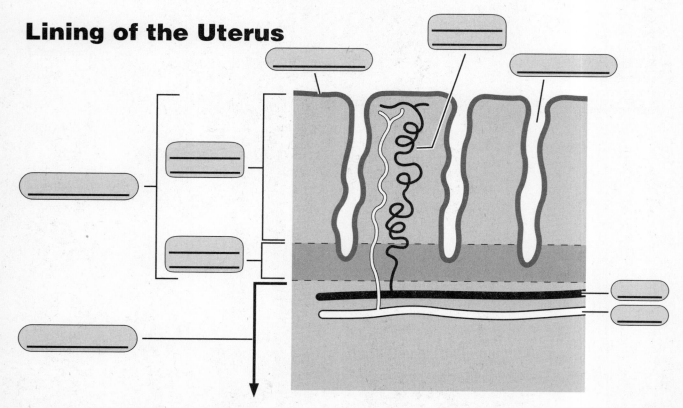

PREGNANT UTERUS

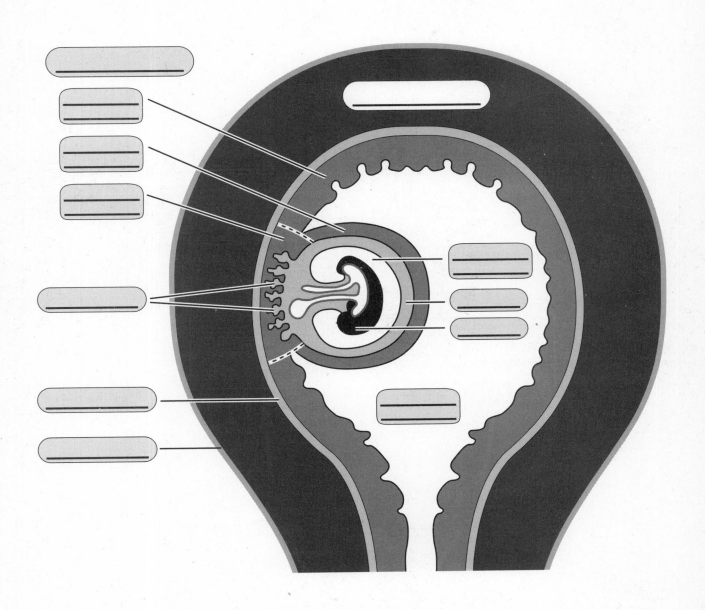

VULVA
Pudendum or External Genitalia

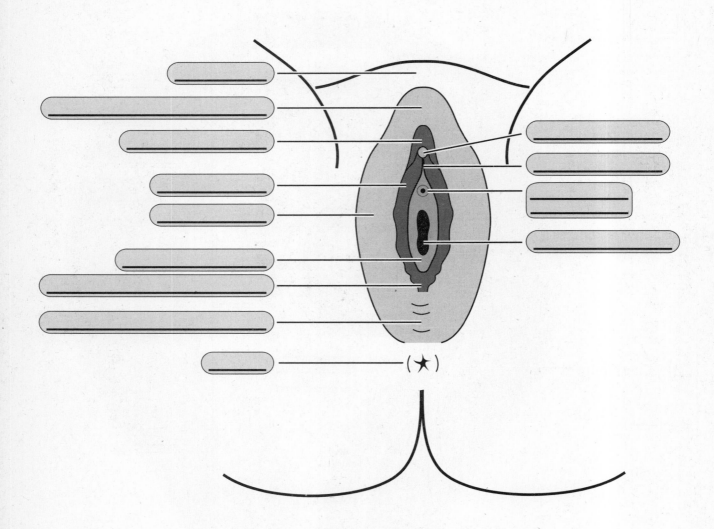

(★)

MAMMARY GLAND

Sagittal Section

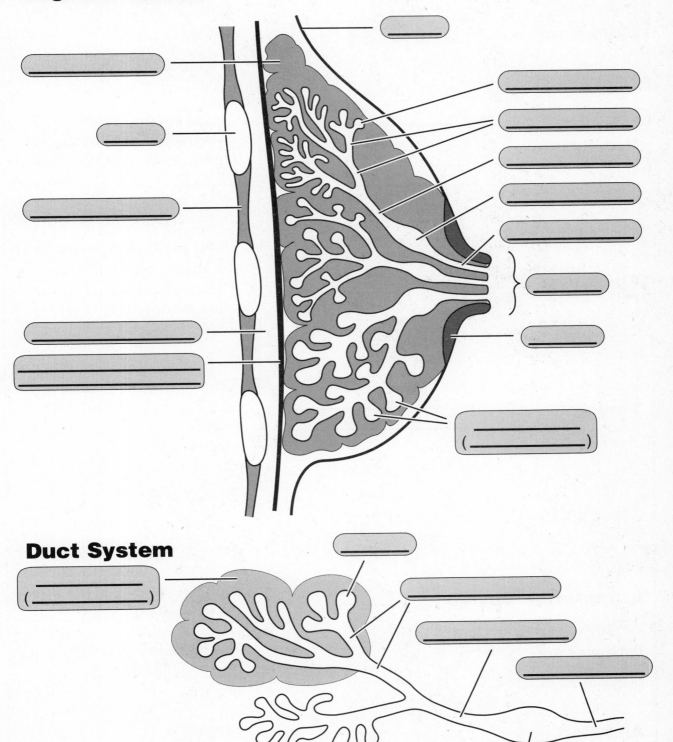

Duct System

BIRTH CONTROL

Methods	Examples	Comments
Hormones	_____ _____ (_____)	Estrogen and progesterone prevent _____development and _____ .
Barriers	_____ _____ _____ _____	_____ are prevented from entering the _____ . Male condoms protect against _____ diseases.
Spermicides	_____ _____ _____ _____ _____ _____	These methods depend upon _____ chemicals. The _____ releases spermicide for up to 24 hours.
Timing	_____ _____	The avoidance of _____ _____ for about 7 days (while a _____ is in the uterine tube).
Sterilization	_____ (_____) _____ (_____)	The severing of each _____ _____ in the male and both _____ in the female.
Intrauterine Device (___)		An object placed in the uterine cavity prevents _____ .
Withdrawal (_____)		The penis is withdrawn from the _____ before _____ occurs.
Abortion		Surgical or _____ removal of the _____ .

FEMALE REPRODUCTIVE CYCLE

Ovarian Cycle

_____ Phase

_____ Phase

Uterine Cycle

_____ Phase

_____ Phase

_____ Phase

Spiral
Arteriole

Straight
Arteriole

Radial
Artery

Stratum _____

Stratum _____

_____

Hormonal Changes

_____

_____

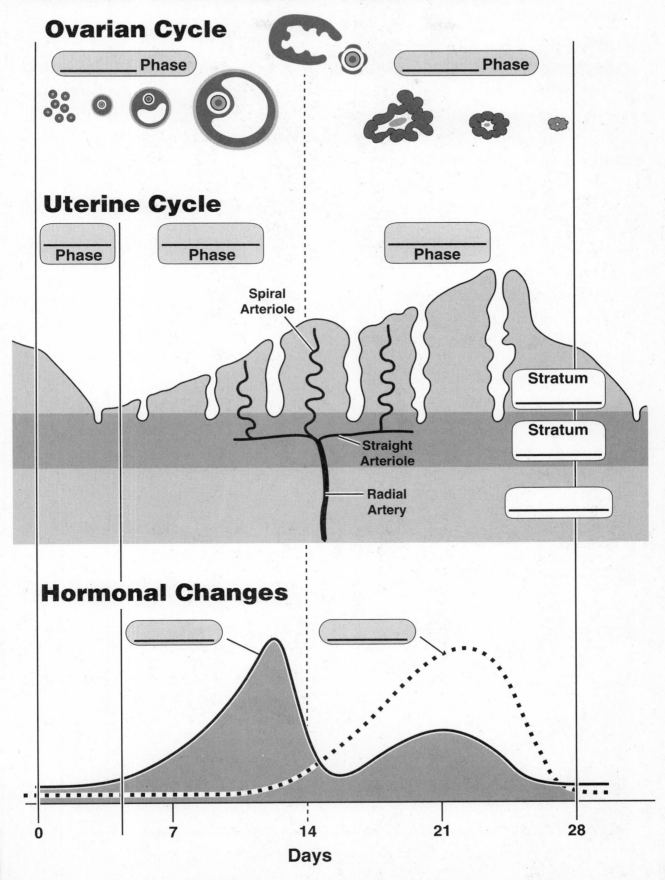

0   7   14   21   28

Days

MENSTRUAL PHASE (days 1 to 5)

Hypothalamus : GnRH released.

Anterior Pituitary : FSH released.

Ovary : Primordial follicles develop into _____ follicles, then into _____ follicles.

Primordial follicles start to develop during the previous cycle (about day 25).

Granulosa (follicular) cells secrete low levels of _____ .

Granulosa cells secrete follicular fluid that fills the follicular cavity (_____)

Uterus : Inner lining of endometrium (_____) sloughs off.

_____ arterioles constrict (due to low levels of estrogen and progesterone).

Cells of the stratum _____ die (due to lack of nourishment).

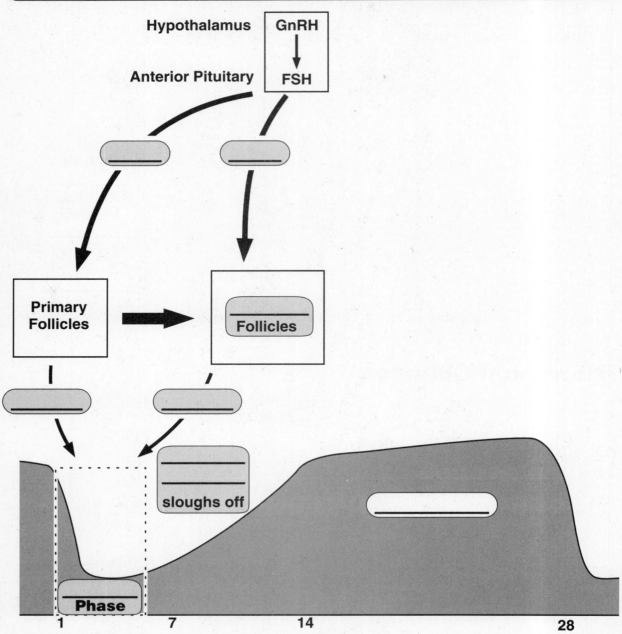

PREOVULATORY PHASE (days 6 to 13)

Hypothalamus : GnRH released.

Anterior Pituitary : _____ released.

_____ levels of estrogen (early part of phase) have a _____ feedback effect.

_____ levels of estrogen (late part of phase) have a _____ feedback effect.

Ovary : Most _____ follicles degenerate (due to decreased FSH secretion).

One _____ secondary follicle matures into a vesicular ovarian follicle.

_____ (follicular) cells secrete _____ .

Uterus : Endometrium thickens; stimulated by _____ .

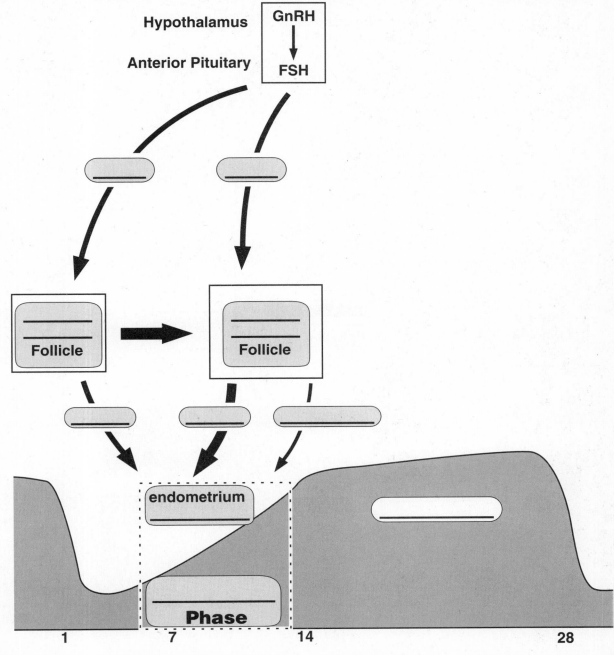

111

OVULATION (day 14)

Hypothalamus : GnRH released; stimulated by high levels of _____ .

Anterior Pituitary : LH released in large quantities (called the _____).

Ovary : _____ triggers ovulation.

_____ follicle ruptures, releasing the _____ .

Uterus : Endometrium thickens; stimulated by high levels of _____ .

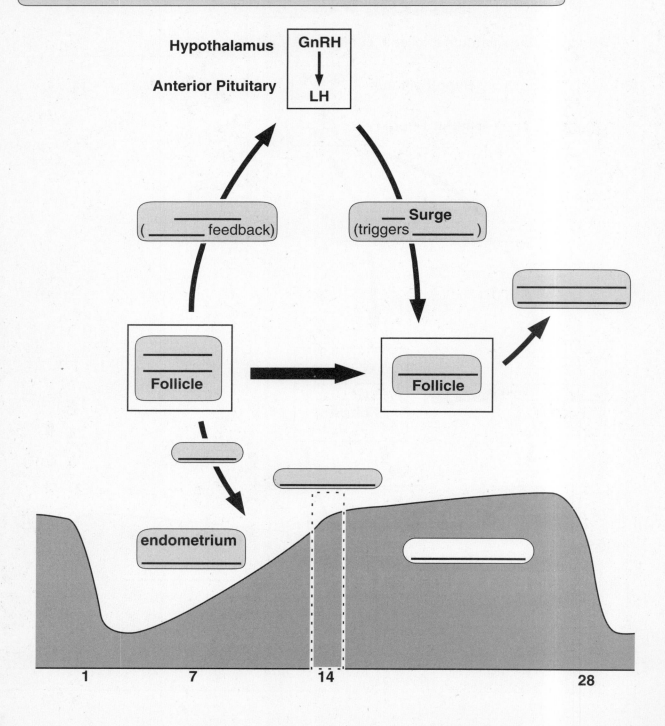

POSTOVULATORY PHASE (days 15 to 28)

Hypothalamus : GnRH released.

Anterior Pituitary : ___ and ___ released.
  High levels of estrogen and progesterone _____ the secretion of LH.
  Low levels of estrogen and progesterone _____ the secretion of FSH.

Ovary : Under the influence of LH, foliicular cells are converted into the _____ .

  The corpus luteum secretes _____ and _____ .

  As LH decreases, the corpus luteum becomes the _____
  (if fertilization has not occurred).

Uterus : Progesterone prepares the endometrium to receive a _____ .

  Decreasing levels of progesterone cause degeneration of the _____
  and initiate a new _____ .

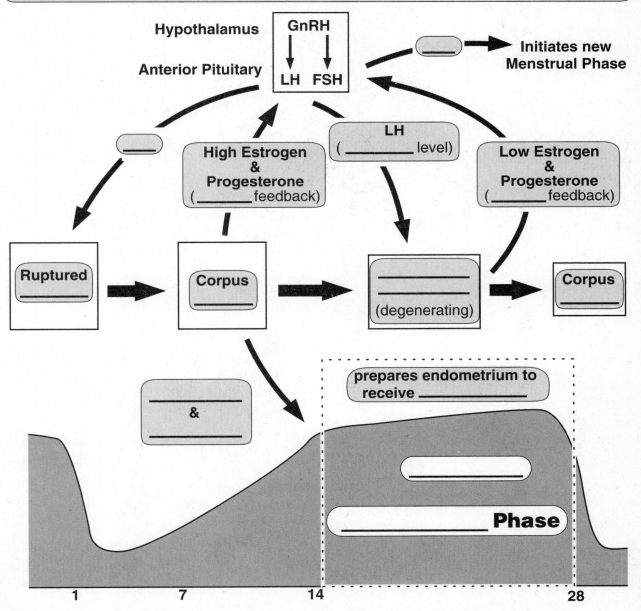

FEMALE REPRODUCTIVE HORMONES

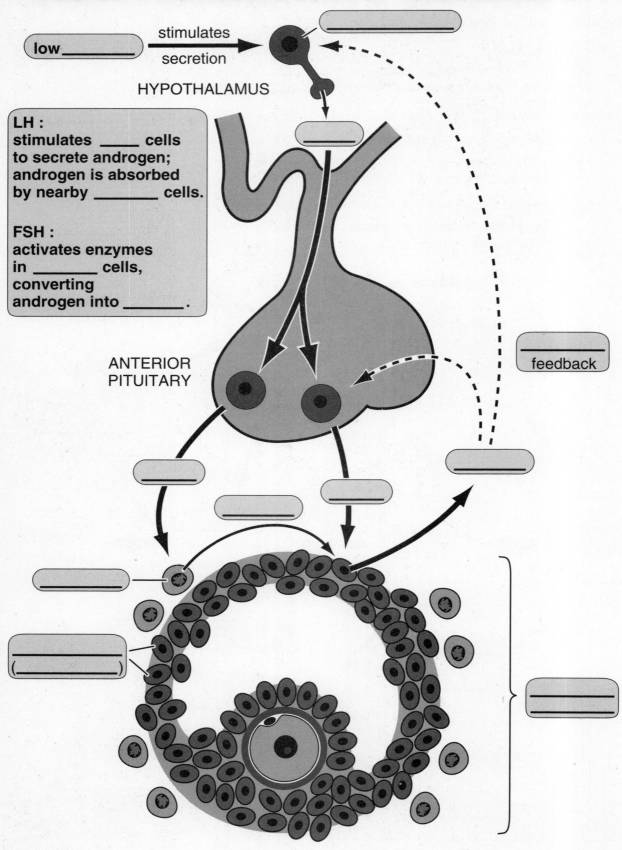

low _____ → stimulates secretion

_____

HYPOTHALAMUS

_____

LH :
stimulates _____ cells
to secrete androgen;
androgen is absorbed
by nearby _____ cells.

FSH :
activates enzymes
in _____ cells,
converting
androgen into _____ .

ANTERIOR
PITUITARY

_____ feedback

_____

_____

_____

_____

_____

_____

_____

DEVELOPMENT

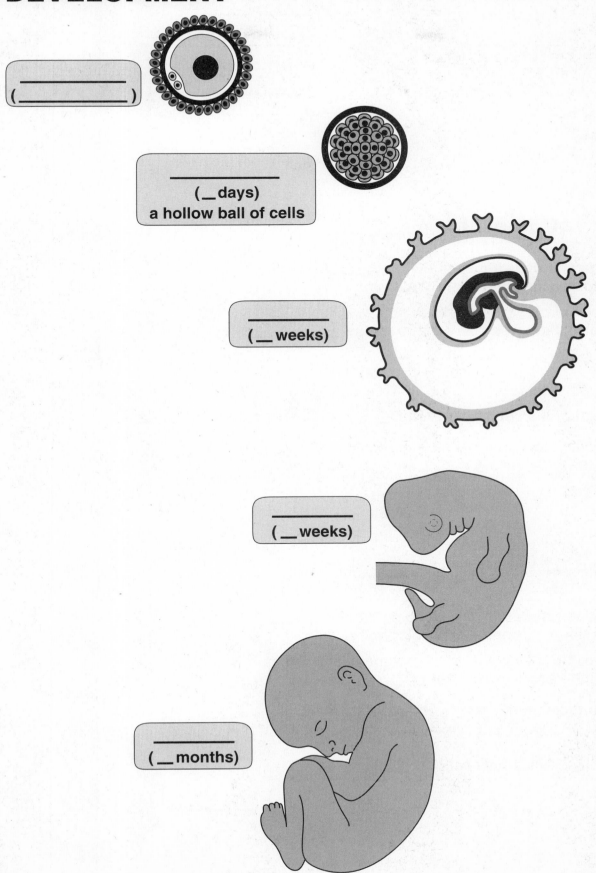

(_____)

_____
(__ days)
a hollow ball of cells

_____
(__ weeks)

_____
(__ weeks)

_____
(__ months)

115

FERTILIZATION

_____ Oocyte
and _____

_____
(_____)

_____
(_____)

_____

_____

Penetration of the _____

One sperm moves between the _____ cells and
binds to species-specific receptors on the _____ .

With the aid of _____ enzymes,
the sperm dissolves and penetrates the _____ .

The head of the sperm fuses with _____ plasma membrane.

Contractile elements in the oocyte draw in the _____ of the
sperm, usually leaving the _____ outside the oocyte.

Fusion of the _____

_____

_____

_____

After penetration, the oocyte completes _____,
forming an _____ and a 2nd polar body.

The nucleus in the ovum and the nucleus in the
head of the sperm are called _____.

The pronuclei fuse, forming a diploid nucleus
called the _____ nucleus.

The diploid cell is now called a _____.

_____

_____

CLEAVAGE AND IMPLANTATION

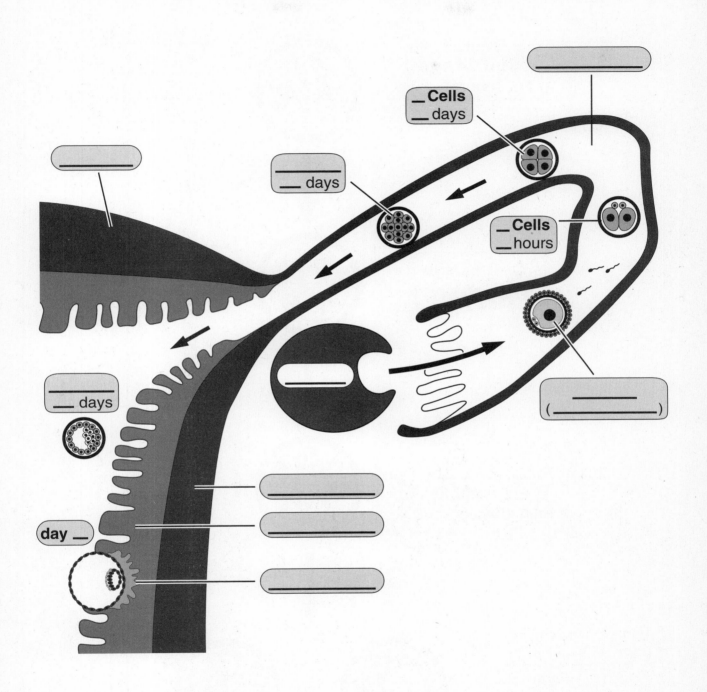

117

CLEAVAGE

Cleavage and the formation of the _____ and _____ .

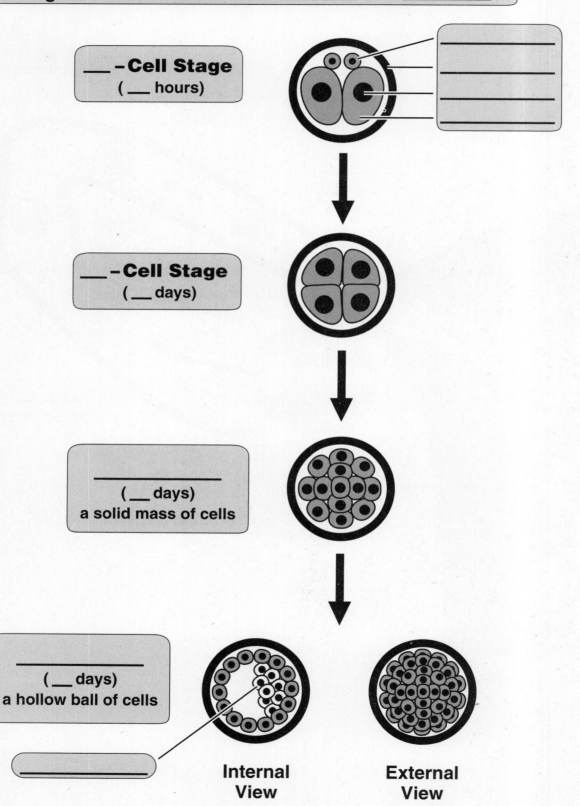

___-Cell Stage
(__ hours)

___-Cell Stage
(__ days)

_____
(__ days)
a solid mass of cells

_____
(__ days)
a hollow ball of cells

Internal
View

External
View

IMPLANTATION

Day 5

_____ is free in the uterine cavity.

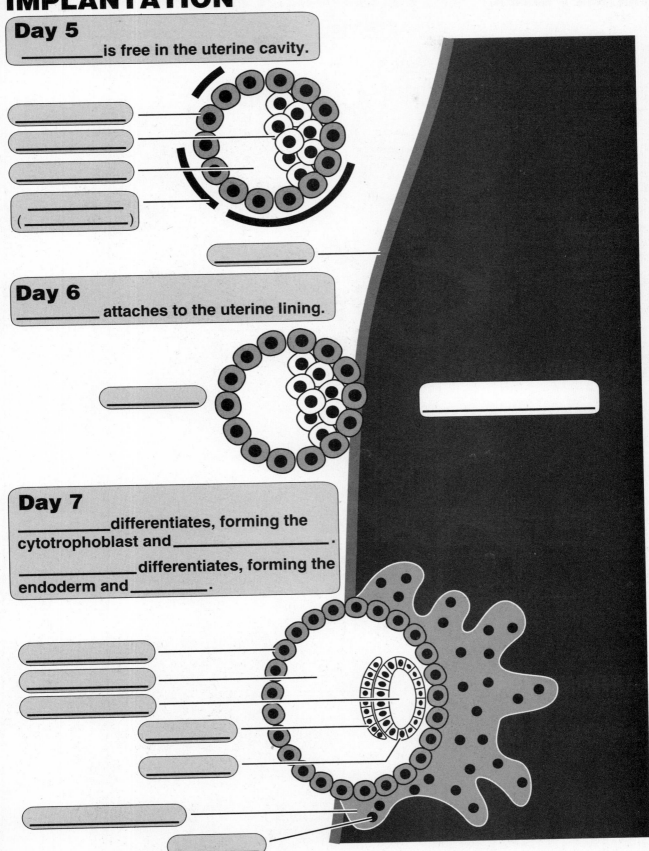

Day 6

_____ attaches to the uterine lining.

Day 7

_____ differentiates, forming the cytotrophoblast and _____ .
_____ differentiates, forming the endoderm and _____ .

EMBRYONIC DEVELOPMENT

The ____ week through the end of the ____ week

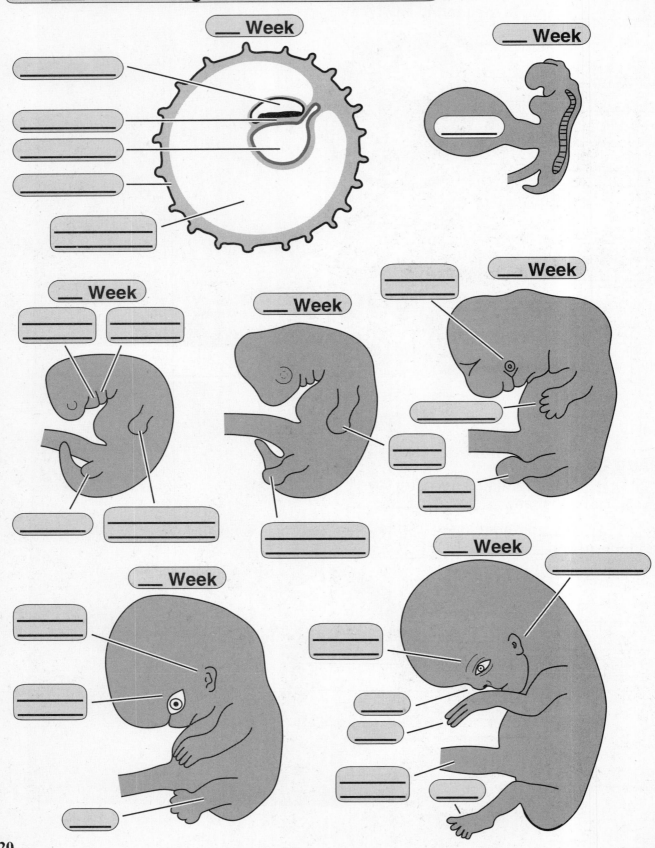

___ Week

___ Week

___ Week

___ Week

___ Week

___ Week

___ Week

120

PRIMARY GERM LAYERS

Simplified Illustration
(individual cells not shown)

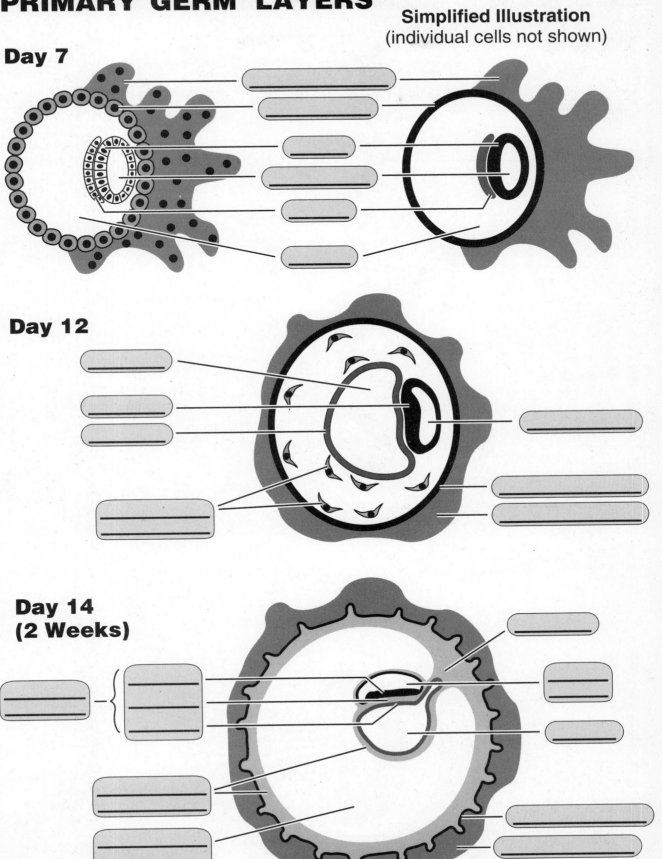

121

EMBRYONIC MEMBRANES

2 Weeks

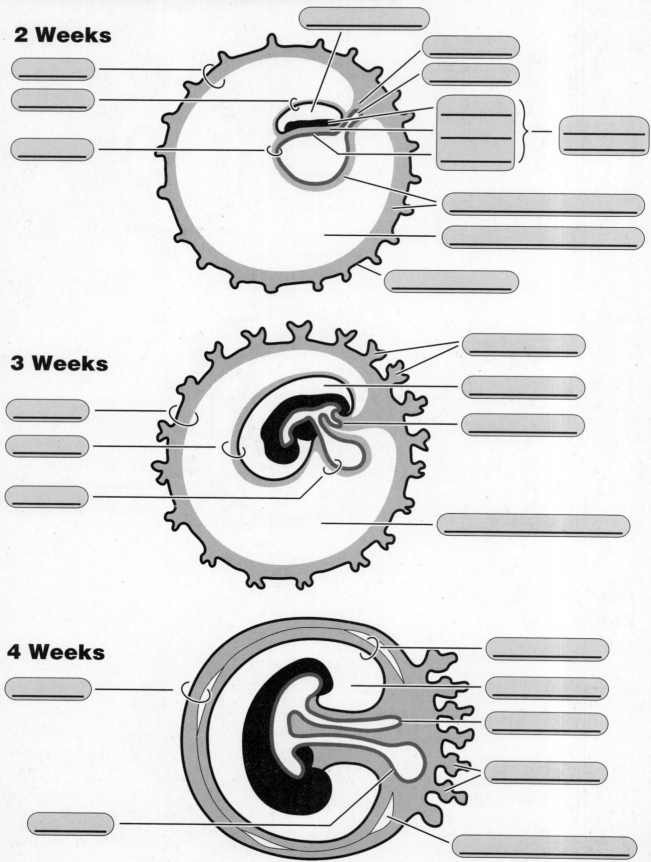

3 Weeks

4 Weeks

PLACENTA AND DECIDUA

Pregnant Uterus

Placenta (detail)

Umbilical arteries not shown.

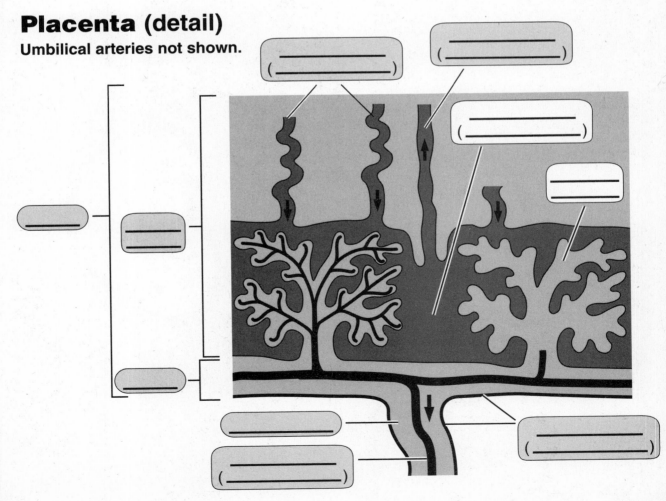

FETAL STAGE

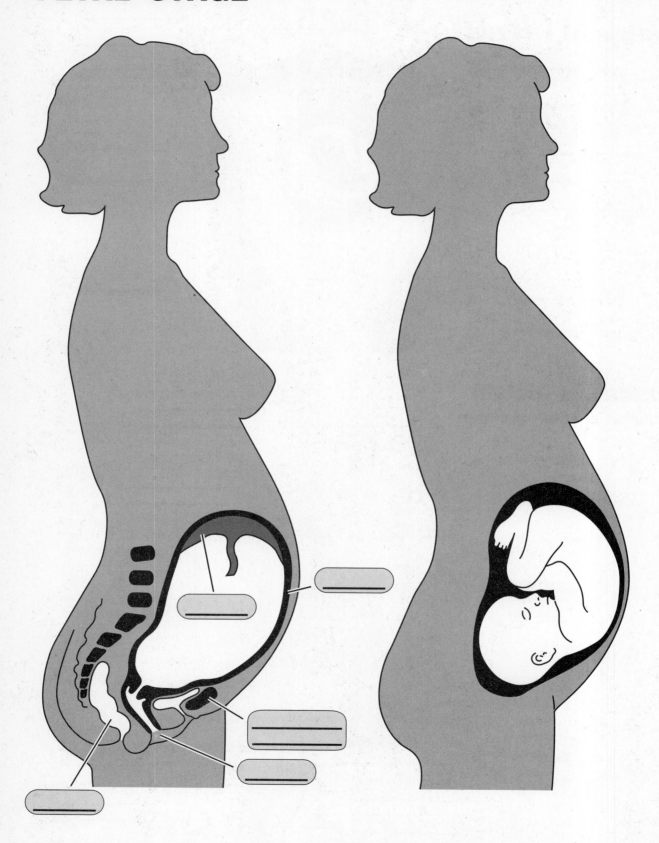

HORMONAL CHANGES

Hormonal Changes During Pregnancy

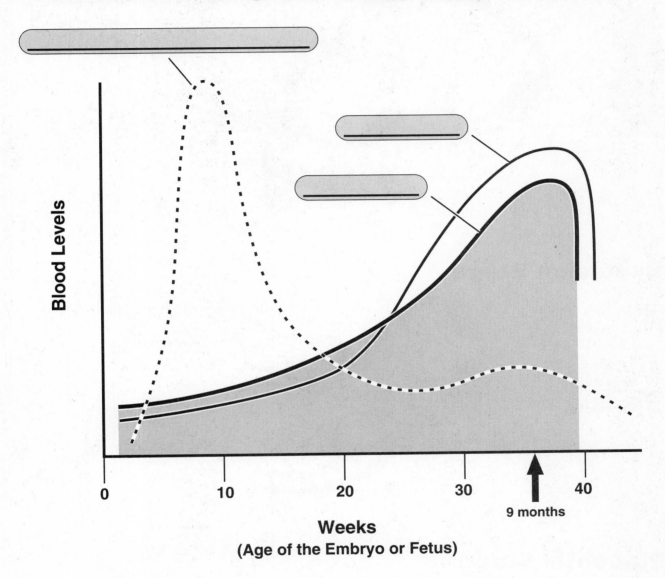

STAGES OF LABOR

Dilation Stage

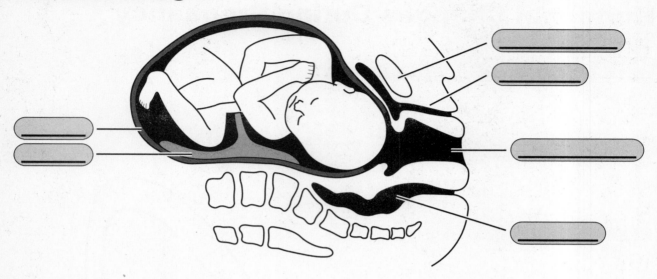

Expulsion Stage

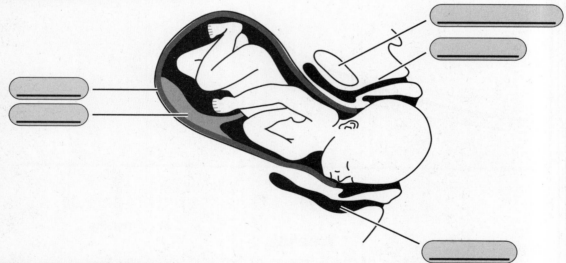

Placental Stage

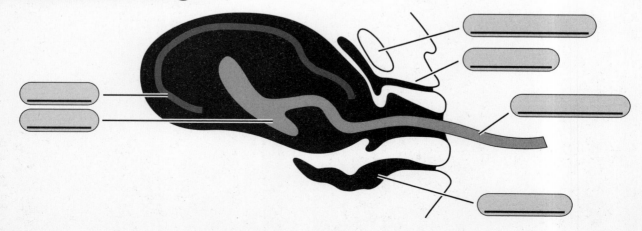

Part III : Terminology

Pronunciation Guide

Pronunciation Key

Accented Syllables

The strongest accented syllable is in capital letters : **dī - ag - NŌ - sis**

Secondary accents are indicated by a prime (′) : **fiz′ - ē - OL - ō - jē**

Vowels

Long vowels are indicated by a horizontal line (macron) above the letter :

ā as in m**a**ke   **ē** as in b**e**   **ī** as in **i**vy   **ō** as in p**o**le

Short vowels are unmarked :

e as in p**e**t   **i** as in p**i**t   **o** as in p**o**t   **u** as in b**u**d

Other Phonetic Symbols

a as in **a**bout   **oo** as in d**o**   **yoo** as in c**u**te   **oy** as in n**oi**se

acrosin **AK - rō - sin**
acrosome **AK - rō - sōm**
aldosterone **al - DA - ster - ōn**
alkaline **AL - ka - līn**
allantois **a - LAN - tō - is**
alveoli **al - VĒ - ō - lī**
amniocentesis **am′ - nē - ō - sen - TĒ - sis**
amnion **AM - nē - on**
amniotic **am′ - nē - OT - ik**
ampulla **am - POOL - la**
anabolic **an - a - BOL - ik**
androgen **AN - drō - jen**
anteflexion **an - tē - FLEK - shun**
antepartum **an - tē - PAR - tum**
arcuate **AR - kyoo - āt**
areola **a - RĒ - ō - la**
atresia **a - TRĒ - zē - a**
autosome **AW - tō - sōm**

Bartholin's **BAR - tō - linz**
blastocele **BLAS - tō - sēl**
blastocyst **BLAS - tō - sist**
blastomere **BLAS - tō - mēr**
bulbourethral **bul′ - bō - yoo - RĒ - thral**

capacitation **ka - pas′ - i - TĀ - shun**
castration **kas - TRĀ - shun**
cavernous urethra **KAV - er - nus yoo - RĒ - thra**
cervical **SER - vi - kul**
cervix **SER - viks**
chorion **KŌ - rē - on**
chorionic **kō′ - rē - ON - ik**
chromatid **KRŌ - ma - tid**
chromosome **KRŌ - mō - sōm**
cleavage **KLĒV - ij**
climacteric **klī - MAK - ter - ik**
clitoris **KLIT - a - ris**
clone **KLŌN**
coelom **SĒ - lum**
coitus interruptus **KŌ - i - tus in - ter - UP- tus**
Cowper's **KOW - perz**
copulation **cop - yoo - LĀ - shun**
corona radiata **kō - RŌ - na rā - dē - A - ta**
corpora cavernosa **KOR - pō - ra ka - ver - NŌ - sa**
corpus albicans **KOR - pus AL - bi - kanz**
corpus hemorrhagicum **KOR - pus hem - or - AJ - i - kum**
corpus luteum **KOR - pus LOO - tē - um**
corpus spongiosum **KOR - pus spun - jē - Ō - sum**
cremaster **krē - MAS - ter**
crura **KROO - ra**
crus **KROOS**
cryptorchidism **krip - TOR - ki - dizm**
cytotrophoblast **sī′ - tō - TRŌF - ō - blast**

dartos **DAR - tōs**
decidua **di - SID - yoo - a**
decidua basalis **di - SID - yoo - a ba - SA - lis**
decidua capsularis **di - SID - yoo - a kap - soo - LA - ris**
decidua parietalis **di - SID - yoo - a par - rī - e - TAL - is**
dihydrotestosterone **dī - hī′ - drō - tes - TOS - ter - ōn**
diploid **DIP - loyd**
dizygotic **dī′ - zī - GOT - ik**
ductus arteriosus **DUK - tus ar - tē - rē - Ō - sus**
ductus deferens **DUK - tus DEF - er - ens**
ductus epididymis **DUK - tus ep - i - DID - i - mus**
ductus venosus **DUK - tus ve - NŌ - sus**

ectoderm　EK-tō-derm

efferent　EF-er-ent

ejaculation　e-jak′-yoo-LĀ-shun

ejaculatory　e-JAK-yoo-la-tō′-rē

embryoblast　EM-brē-ō-blast′

embryology　em′-brē-OL-ō-jē

embryonic　em′-brē-ON-ik

endocrinocyte　en′-dō-KRIN-ō-sīt′

endoderm　EN-dō-derm

endometrial　en′-dō-MĒ-trē-al

endometrium　en′-dō-MĒ-trē-um

epididymis　ep′-i-DID-i-mis

estrogen　ES-tro-jen

Fallopian　fal-LŌ-pē-an

fetal　FĒ-tal

fetus　FĒ-tus

fibrinogen　fī-BRIN-ō-jen

fibrinolysin　fī-brin-OL-i-sin

fimbria　FIM-brē-a

fimbriae　FIM-brē-ē

flaccid　FLAS-sid

follicle　FOL-i-kul

follicular　fō-LIK-yoo-lar

foramen ovale　fō-RĀ-men ō-VAL-ē

fornix　FOR-niks

frenulum　FREN-yoo-lum

fructose　FRUK-tōs

fundus　FUN-dus

gamete　GAM-ēt

gameteogenesis　gam′-e-tō-JEN-e-sis

gastrulation　gas′-troo-LĀ-shun

genetalia　jen′-i-TĀL-ya

germinal　JER-mi-nal

gestation　jes-TĀ-shun

glans clitoris　GLANZ KLIT-a-ris

glans penis　GLANZ PĒ-nis

gonad　GŌ-nad

gonadotropin　gō′-nad-ō-TRŌ-pin

Graafian　GRAF-ē-an

granulosa　gran-yoo-LŌ-sa

gynecology　gī′-ne-KOL-ō-jē

haploid　HAP-loyd

hilum　HĪ-lum

hilus　HĪ-lus

homologous　hō-MOL-ō-gus

homologue　HOM-ō-log

hyaluronic　hī′-a-loo-RON-ik

hyaluronidase　hī′-a-loo-RON-i-dās

hymen　HĪ-men

iliac　IL-ē-ak

infundibulum　in′-fun-DIB-yoo-lum

inguinal　IN-gwin-al

inhibin　in-HIB-in

interstitial　in′-ter-STISH-al

intervillous　in-ter-VIL-us

isthmus　IS-mus

labia majora　LĀ-bē-a ma-JŌ-ra

labia minora　LĀ-bē-a mī-NŌ-ra

labium majus　LĀ-bē-um MĀ-jus

labium minus　LĀ-bē-um MĪ-nus

lactation　lak-TĀ-shun

lactiferous　lak-TIF-er-us

lactogenic　lak-tō-JEN-ik

Leydig　LĪ-dig

ligation　lī-GĀ-shun

Littre　LĒ-tra

lobule　LOB-yool

luteal　LOO-tē-al

luteinizing　LOO-tē-in′-īz-ing

mammography　mam-OG-ra-fē

meiosis　mī-Ō-sis

membranous　MEM-bra-nus

menarche　me-NAR-kē

menopause　MEN-ō-pawz

menses　MEN-sēz

menstrual　MEN-stroo-al

menstruation　men′-stroo-Ā-shun

mesoderm　MEZ-ō-derm

mesovarium　mez′-ō-VAR-ē-um

mitosis　mī-TŌ-sis

mittelschmerz　MIT-el-shmārts

monozygotic　mon′-ō-zī-GOT-ik

mons pubis　MONZ PYOO-bis

morula　MOR-yoo-la

mucosa　myoo-KŌ-sa

mucous　MYOO-kus

mucus　MYOO-kus

muscularis　MUS-kyoo-la′-ris

myoepithelial　mī′-ō-ep′-i-THĒ-lē-al

myoid　MĪ-oyd

myometrium　mī′-ō-MĒ-trē-um

navel　NĀ-vel

neonatal　nē′-ō-NĀ-tal

obstetrics　ob-STET-riks

oocyte　Ō-ō-sīt

oogenesis　ō′-ō-JEN-e-sis

oogonia　ō′-ō-GŌ-nē-a

oogonium　ō′-ō-GŌ-nē-um

orgasm　OR-gazm

os　OS

ova   Ō-va
ovarian   ō-VAR-ē-an
ovary   Ō-var-ē
oviduct   Ō-vi-dukt
ovulation   ō-vyoo-LĀ-shun
ovum   Ō-vum

paraurethral   per'-a-yoo-RĒ-thral
parturition   par'-too-RISH-un
pelvic   PEL-vik
penis   PĒ-nis
perimetrium   per'-i-MĒ-trē-um
perineum   per'-i-NĒ-um
peristalsis   per'-i-STAL-sis
placenta   pla-SEN-ta
placental   pla-SEN-tal
polyspermy   pol'-ē-SPER-mē
postovulatory   pōst-OV-yoo-la-tor-ē
preovulatory   prē-OV-yoo-la-tor-ē
prepuce   PRĒ-pyoos
primordial   prī-MOR-dē-al
progesterone   prō-JES-te-rōn
prolactin   prō-LAK-tin
proliferation   prō-lif'-er-Ā-shun
proliferative   prō-LIF-er-a-tiv
pronuclei   prō-NOO-klē-ī
pronucleus   prō-NOO-klē-us
prostaglandin   pros'-ta-GLAN-din
prostate   PROS-tāt
prostatic   pros-TAT-ik
puberty   PYOO-ber-tē
pubic symphysis   PYOO-bik SIM-fi-sis
pudendum   pyoo-DEN-dum

rectouterine   rek'-tō-YOO-ter-in
relaxin   rē-LAK-sin
rete testis   RĒ-tē TES-tis
reticulum   re-TIK-yoo-lum
retroflexion   re-trō-FLEK-shun
ruga   ROO-ga
rugae   ROO-jē

scrotum   SKRŌ-tum
secretory   si-KRĒ-to-rē
segmentation   seg'-men-TĀ-shun
semen   SĒ-men
seminal plasmin   SEM-i-nal PLAZ-min
seminiferous   sem'-i-NI-fer-us
serosa   ser-Ō-sa
Sertoli   ser-TŌ-lē
Skene's   SKĒNZ
spermatic   sper-MAT-ik
spermatid   SPER-ma-tid
spermatocyte   SPER-ma-tō-sīt'

spermatogenesis   sper'-ma-tō-JEN-e-sis
spermatogonia   sper'-ma-tō-GŌ-nē-a
spermatogonium   sper'-ma-tō-GŌ-nē-um
spermatozoa   sper'-ma-tō-ZŌ-a
spermatozoon   sper'-ma-tō-ZŌ-on
spermiation   sper-mē-Ā-shun
spermicide   SPER-mi-sīd'
spermiogenesis   sper'-mē-ō-JEN-e-sis
sphincter   SFINGK-ter
stratum basalis   STRĀ-tum ba-SAL-is
stratum functionalis   STRĀ-tum funk'-shun-AL-is
stroma   STRŌ-ma
sustentacular   sus'-ten-TAK-yoo-lar
synapsis   sin-AP-sis
syncytiotrophoblast   sin-sīt'-ē-ō-TRŌF-ō-blast
syngamy   SING-ga-mē

testes   TES-tēz
testis   TES-tis
testosterone   tes-TOS-te-rōn
tetrad   TE-trad
trophoblast   TRŌF-ō-blast
tubule   TOO-byool
tunica albuginea   TOO-ni-ka al'-byoo-JIN-ē-a
tunica vaginalis   TOO-ni-ka va-jin-AL-is

umbilical   um-BIL-i-kul
umbilicus   um-BIL-i-kus
urethra   yoo-RĒ-thra
urethral   yoo-RĒ-thral
urogenital   yoo'-rō-JEN-i-tal
uterine   YOO-ter-in
uterosacral   yoo'-ter-ō-SĀ-kral
uterus   YOO-te-rus

vagina   va-JĪ-na
vaginal   VA-ji-nal
vas deferens   VAS DEF-e-rens
vasectomy   vas-EK-tō-mē
vesicle   VES-i-kul
vesicouterine   ves'-i-kō-YOO-ter-in
vesicular   ve-SIK-yoo-lar
vestibular   ves-TIB-yoo-lar
vestibule   VES-ti-byool
vulva   VUL-va

Wharton's   HWAR-tunz
womb   WOOM

zona pellucida   ZŌ-na pe-LOO-si-da
zygote   ZĪ-gōt

Glossary of Terms

Accessory sex glands   The glands (in the male) that secrete most of the liquid portion of semen. They include the two seminal vesicles, the prostate gland, and the two bulbourethral glands.

Acrosin An enzyme produced by the acrosome of a sperm that stimulates sperm motility and migration.

Acrosome   A dense granule in the head of a spermatozoon. It contains enzymes that facilitate the penetration of a spermatozoon into a secondary oocyte.

Afterbirth   *See* Placenta.

Alkaline solution   A solution that contains more hydroxyl ions (OH^-) than hydrogen ions (H^+); a pH greater than 7. The semen is slightly alkaline (pH 7.20–7.60). Also called a *basic solution*.

Allantois   One of the four embryonic membranes. It serves as an early site for blood formation.

Alveolus   (plural: alveoli)   A hollow or cavity. A milk-secreting gland in the breasts. An air sac in the lungs.

Amniocentesis The examination of embryonic cells sloughed off into the amniotic fluid.

Amnion   One of the four embryonic membranes. It is a transparent membrane that forms a fluid-filled sac surrounding the embryo (or fetus). Also called the *amniotic membrane* and *bag of waters*.

Amniotic cavity   The fluid-filled cavity between the embryo (or fetus) and the amnion.

Amniotic fluid   The fluid in the amniotic cavity.

Amniotic membrane   *See* Amnion.

Ampulla   A saclike dilation of a canal.

Anabolic hormones   Hormones that stimulate anabolism (especially the synthesis of proteins).

Androgen   A collective term for male sex hormones.

Anteflexion   The normal forward curvature of the uterus.

Antepartum   Occurring to the mother before childbirth.

Antrum   *See* Follicular cavity.

Arcuate arteries   Arteries arranged in a circular fashion around the uterus. They are branches of the uterine arteries.

Areola   The pigmented ring around the nipple of the breast.

Ateriole A small (almost microscopic) blood vessel between an artery and a capillary.

Atresia   The degeneration of an ovarian follicle before it reaches maturity.

Autosome   Any chromosome other than the pair of sex chromosomes (the X and Y chromosomes).

Bag of waters   *See* Amnion.

Bartholin's glands   *See* Greater vestibular glands.

Basal layer   *See* Stratum basalis.

Basement membrane   A layer of extracellular material that attaches the epithelial tissue to the underlying connective tissue. A basement membrane surrounds each seminiferous tubule in the testes.

Basic solution   *See* Alkaline solution.

Blastocele   The fluid-filled cavity in the blastocyst.

Blastocyst A hollow ball of cells that forms about the fifth day after fertilization. It consists of an outer covering of cells (the trophoblast), an inner cell mass, and a fluid-filled cavity (the blastocele).

Blastomere   One of the cells formed by cleavage of the fertilized ovum.

Blood-testis barrier   A barrier formed by the tight junctions between adjacent sustentacular (Sertoli) cells in the seminiferous tubules of the testes. It prevents an immune response against antigens produced by developing spermatozoa.

Body of the penis   The free, pendulous part of the penis.

Body of the uterus   The expanded, superior two-thirds of the uterus.

Broad ligament   A double layer of parietal peritoneum that attaches the uterus to the side of the pelvic cavity.

Bulb of the penis   The expanded portion at the base of the corpus spongiosum (the erectile tissue that surrounds the spongy urethra in the penis).

Bulb of the vestibule   Two elongated masses of erectile tissue on either side of the vaginal orifice. Homologous to the corpus spongiosum of the male penis.

Bulbourethral gland   One of a pair of glands located inferior to the prostate gland. It secretes an alkaline fluid into the spongy urethra during ejaculation. Also called *Cowper's gland*.

Capacitation   The functional changes that sperm undergo in the female reproductive tract that allow them (give them the capacity) to fertilize a secondary oocyte.

Cardinal ligaments   Ligaments that extend laterally from the vagina and the uterine cervix. A continuation of the broad ligaments on each side of the uterus and vagina. Also called the *lateral cervical ligaments*.

Castration   Removal of the testes.

Cavernous urethra   *See* Spongy urethra.

Cervical canal   The space inside the cervix of the uterus.

Cervical mucus   A substance secreted by cells in the mucous lining (mucosa) of the uterine cervix. It is a mixture of water, glycoprotein, lipids, enzymes, and inorganic salts.

Cervical cap   A device used for birth control; it is made of latex and fits over the cervix of the uterus.

Cervix   Neck; any constricted portion of an organ. For example, the lower cylindrical part of the uterus.

Childbirth   *See* Labor.

Chorion   One of the four embryonic membranes. It is derived from mesoderm and the outer layer of cells of the blastocyst (the trophoblast). It surrounds the amnion and eventually fuses with it. It forms the embryonic portion of the placenta.

Chorionic villi   Fingerlike projections of the chorion that extend into the lining of the uterus (endometrium), forming the placenta. Fetal blood vessels fill the internal spaces of the chorionic villi.

Chromatid   One of a pair of identical strands of DNA joined by a centromere; the result of chromosome replication. During mitosis, each chromatid moves to a different daughter cell and becomes a chromosome.

Chromosome   One of the 46 small, dark-staining bodies that appear in the nucleus of a cell during cell division. Each chromosome contains a single DNA molecule and associated proteins.

Chromosome number The number of chromosomes in a cell. All body cells contain the diploid number (46 chromosomes); gametes (sperm and ova) contain the haploid number (23 chromosomes).

Circumcision Surgical removal of the prepuce (foreskin), the fold of skin over the glans penis of the male.

Cleavage The rapid cell divisions (mitosis) following the fertilization of a secondary oocyte. The resulting cells are called blastomeres.

Climacteric Cessation of the reproductive cycle in the female; decreased activity of the testes in the male.

Climax The period of greatest intensity. The climax during sexual excitement is called *orgasm*.

Clitoris An erectile organ of the female that is homologous to the male penis. It is located at the anterior junction of the labia minora.

Clone A population of identical cells.

Clotting enzymes Enzymes secreted by the prostate gland. They act on fibrinogen, secreted by the seminal vesicles, causing the semen to coagulate in the vagina.

Coitus *See* Sexual intercourse.

Coitus interruptus A birth control method. The withdrawal of the penis from the vagina before ejaculation. Also called *withdrawal*.

Conception Fertilization of the ovum and the formation of a zygote; the onset of pregnancy.

Condom A device used for birth control. A latex covering placed over the penis.

Confinement *See* Labor.

Contraceptive An agent that prevents (or diminishes the likelihood of) conception.

Contraceptive sponge A birth control method. A polyurethane sponge that contains a spermicide (nonoxynol–9).

Cooper's ligaments *See* Suspensory ligaments.

Copulation *See* Sexual intercourse.

Corona Crown. A crownlike or encircling structure.

Corona of glans penis The margin of the glans penis.

Corona radiata Several layers of granulosa (follicle) cells that remain attached to a secondary oocyte after ovulation.

Corpora cavernosa (singular: corpus cavernosum) Two masses of spongy erectile tissue in the penis.

Corpus Body. The principal part of any organ; any mass or body.

Corpus albicans A structure that replaces the corpus luteum in the ovary during the final days of the menstrual cycle. It consists of white fibrous tissue.

Corpus hemorrhagicum An ovarian follicle or corpus luteum that contains a blood clot.

Corpus luteum A yellow endocrine gland in the ovary. It develops from a ruptured mature follicle soon after ovulation. It secretes estrogen, progesterone, relaxin, and inhibin.

Corpus spongiosum A single mass of spongy erectile tissue in the penis. Its expanded base is called the bulb of the penis. Its distal end forms the tip of the penis and is called the glans penis.

Cowper's gland *See* Bulbourethral gland.

Cremaster muscle A band of skeletal muscle that is part of the spermatic cord and is a continuation of the internal oblique muscle of the abdominal wall. It elevates the testes during sexual arousal and on exposure to cold.

Crossing-over The exchange of a portion of one chromatid with another in a tetrad during meiosis I. As a result, two chromatids that had been identical become genetically different. This greatly increases the genetic variability of the gametes (sperm or ova) that are formed.

Crura of the penis The separated and tapered portions of the corpora cavernosa of the penis.

Cryptorchidism The condition of undescended testes.

Cytoplasmic bridge A cytoplasmic strand that connects two adjacent cells. During the meiosis of spermatocytes (in the seminiferous tubules) the daughter cells are connected by cytoplasmic bridges.

Cytotrophoblast One of the two layers of cells that differentiate from the trophoblast just before implantation. The cytotrophoblast consists of well-defined cells (*cyto* = cell). The other layer is called the syncytiotrophoblast (the nuclei are not separated by plasma membranes).

Dartos The muscle under the skin of the scrotum.

Daughter cell A cell that results from a cell division. The original cell is called the parent cell.

Decidua That portion of the endometrium (of the uterus) that is shed after childbirth. It includes all but the deepest layer (stratum basalis) of the endometrium.

Decidua basalis The portion of the endometrium that underlies the embryo (or fetus).

Decidua capsularis The portion of the endometrium between the embryo (fetus) and the uterine cavity.

Decidua parietalis The portion of the endometrium that lines the uterine cavity; the portion that is not the decidua basalis or the decidua capsularis.

Deciduous Falling off or being shed seasonally.

Deep Away from the surface of the body.

Deep inguinal ring A slitlike opening in the transversus abdominus muscle through which the spermatic cord passes. The origin of the inguinal canal.

Delivery *See* Labor.

DHT *See* Dihydrotestosterone.

Diaphragm A device used for birth control; a rubber dome–shaped device that fits over the cervix of the uterus.

Dihydrotestosterone (DHT) A hormone (an androgen) derived from testosterone. It stimulates the male pattern of development before birth, the development of secondary sex characteristics, and anabolism (protein synthesis).

Diploid Having the number of chromosomes found in all cells except gametes (sperm and ova). Symbolized 2*n*.

Dizygotic twins Twins produced from the independent release of two ova and the subsequent fertilization of each by different spermatozoa. Also called *fraternal twins*.

Dominant primary follicle The primary follicle that contains a primary oocyte that completes meiosis I, producing a polar body and a secondary oocyte. Several primary follicles develop from primordial follicles each month, but most of these follicles degenerate (atresia). Only the dominant follicle continues to develop.

Duct A tube or passageway with well-defined walls.

Ductus arteriosus A passageway that connects the pulmonary trunk with the aorta. Present only in the fetus. It shunts blood directly from the right ventricle to the aorta, bypassing the lungs, which are nonfunctional in the fetus.

Ductus deferens The duct that carries spermatozoa from the ductus epididymis (outside each testis) to the ejaculatory duct, which leads into the prostatic urethra. Also called *vas deferens* and *seminal duct*.

Ductus epididymis A highly coiled tube inside the epididymis. Spermatozoa become fully mature and are stored in the ductus epididymis until ejaculation.

Ductus venosus A branch of the umbilical vein that bypasses the liver and carries oxygenated blood directly to the inferior vena cava. During fetal development, the liver is nonfunctional, except for the production of red blood cells.

Ectoderm One of the three primary germ layers. It gives rise to the nervous system and the epidermis of the skin.

Efferent duct A coiled tube that transports spermatozoa from the rete testis to the ductus epididymis.

Egg *See* Ovum.

Ejaculation The ejection of semen from the penis. It has two phases: (1) emission (the movement of semen into the urethra) and (2) expulsion (the propulsion of semen out of the urethra at the time of orgasm).

Ejaculatory duct A short tube about one inch long that connects the ampulla of the ductus deferens to the prostatic urethra.

Ejection In the mammary glands, ejection refers to the movement of milk from the alveoli into the ducts. The hormone oxytocin (OT) stimulates myoepithelial cells surrounding the walls of the alveoli to contract, compressing the alveoli and ejecting milk into the ducts, where it can be suckled.

Embryo The developing organism from the end of the 2nd week to the end of the 8th week. The appearance of the embryonic disc (the three primary germ layers) at the end of the second week marks the beginning of embryonic development.

Embryoblast *See* Inner cell mass.

Embryology The scientific study of the embryo.

Embryonic Pertaining to the embryo.

Embryonic disc The embryo at its earliest stage of development. Consists of three layers of primary germ cells: ectoderm, mesoderm, and endoderm. Appears at about the fourteenth day after fertilization.

Embryonic period The period of development from the end of the 2nd week to the end of the 8th week. Sometimes more generally defined as the first two months of development.

Emission The movement of semen into the urethra; the first phase of ejaculation.

Endoderm One of the primary germ layers. It gives rise to the lining of the gastrointestinal tract, respiratory tract, and urinary bladder.

Endometrium The mucous membrane lining the uterus. It is divided into two layers: (1) the stratum functionalis, which is shed during menstruation, and (2) the stratum basalis, which gives rise to a new stratum functionalis after each menstruation.

Epididymis A comma-shaped structure that lies along the posterior border of each testis and contains the ductus epididymis.

Erection The rigid and enlarged state of the penis (or clitoris) resulting from the engorgement of the spongy erectile tissue with blood.

Estrogen A group of steroid hormones. The major estrogen secreted by the granulosa (follicle) cells of the ovaries is called estradiol. The major estrogen secreted by the placenta during pregnancy is called estriol.

External os The narrow opening between the cervical canal and the vagina.

External urethral orifice The opening of the urethra (male and female) to the exterior.

Extraembryonic coelom A cavity that surrounds the embryonic disc, amniotic cavity, and yolk sac during the third week of embryonic development.

Fallopian tube *See* Uterine tube.

Female condom *See* Vaginal pouch.

Female reproductive cycle A general term for the ovarian and uterine cycles, the hormonal changes that accompany them, and the cyclic changes in the breasts and cervix.

Fertilization Penetration of a secondary oocyte by a spermatozoon and the subsequent union of the nuclei (pronuclei) of the sperm and ovum.

Fetal Pertaining to the fetus.

Fetus The developing organism from the beginning of the 3rd month until birth, usually at the end of the 9th month.

Fibrinolysin An enzyme secreted by the prostate gland. It dissolves coagulated (clotted) semen in the vagina.

Fimbriae (singular: fimbria) Fingerlike projections of the infundibulum (the funnel-shaped distal end of each uterine tube).

Flaccid Relaxed, flabby, or soft. Lacking muscle tone.

Follicle A small secretory sac or cavity. An ovarian follicle is a cluster of granulosa (follicle) cells surrounding an oocyte (developing ovum).

Follicle-stimulating hormone (FSH) A hormone secreted by the anterior pituitary gland. It initiates the development of follicles in females and stimulates sperm production in males.

Follicular cavity The fluid-filled cavity in a developing ovarian follicle. Also called the *antrum*.

Follicular cells *See* Granulosa cells.

Follicular phase A phase of the ovarian cycle. The first fourteen days of the menstrual cycle, when follicles are growing and developing.

Foramen A passage or opening.

Foramen ovale An opening in the septum of the fetal heart. It allows blood to pass directly from the right ventricle to the left ventricle, bypassing the lungs (which are nonfunctional in the fetus).

Foreskin *See* Prepuce.

Fornix An arch or fold. The recess around the cervix of the uterus where it protrudes into the vagina.

Fraternal twins *See* Dizygotic twins.

Frenulum A small fold or mucous membrane that connects two parts and limits movement. The labia minora form the frenulum of the clitoris just posterior to the glans clitoris.

Fructose A sugar present in the fluid secreted by the seminal vesicles. It provides sperm with an energy source.

Functional layer *See* Stratum functionalis.

FSH *See* Follicle-stimulating hormone.

Fundus The part of a hollow organ farthest from the opening. The dome-shaped portion of the uterus located above the entrance of the uterine tubes is called the fundus.

Gamete A male or female reproductive cell; a spermatozoon (sperm) or ovum (egg).

Gametogenesis The cell divisions that result in the production of gametes (spermatozoa or ova).

Gastrulation   The movements of cells in the developing organism that lead to the formation of the primary germ layers (ectoderm, mesoderm, and endoderm).

Gene   The basic hereditary unit. A portion of a DNA molecule. The chromosomes of each cell contain a total of about 100,000 genes.

Genetics   The study of heredity.

Genitalia   External and internal reproductive organs.

Germinal epithelium   A layer of epithelium that covers the surface of the ovary.

Gestation   The period of development from the time of fertilization of the ovum until birth. In humans, the gestation period is about 266 days.

Glans clitoris   The exposed portion of the clitoris.

Glans penis   The distal end of the corpus spongiosum. It forms the slightly enlarged tip of the penis.

GnRH   *See* Gonadotropin-releasing hormone.

Golgi complex   An organelle in the cytoplasm of cells consisting of four to eight membranous sacs. During the formation of a sperm from a spermatid, the Golgi complex develops into an enzyme-containing structure (acrosome).

Gonad   A gland that produces gametes and hormones; the ovary in the female and the testis in the male.

Gonadotropin   A hormone that regulates the functions of the gonads. Examples are follicle-stimulating hormone (FSH) and luteinizing hormone (LH).

Gonadotropin-releasing hormone (GnRH)   A hormone secreted by the hypothalamus that stimulates the release of gonadotropins (FSH and LH) by the anterior pituitary gland.

Graafian follicle   *See* Vesicular ovarian follicle.

Granulosa cells   The cells that surround an oocyte, forming a follicle. They are located in the ovaries and secrete estrogen. Also called *follicular cells.*

Greater vestibular glands   A pair of glands on either side of the vaginal orifice that are homologous to the male bulbourethral glands. They open by ducts into a groove between the hymen and the labia minora and secrete mucus that supplements lubrication during sexual intercourse. Also called *Bartholin's glands.*

Gynecology   A branch of medicine that deals with disorders of the female reproductive system.

Haploid   The number of chromosomes (23) present in gametes; half the number present in all other cells of the body. Symbolized by *n.*

hCG   *See* Human chorionic gonadotropin.

hCS   *See* Human chorionic somatomammotropin.

Hilum   *See* Hilus.

Hilus   An area, depression, or pit where blood vessels and nerves enter and leave an organ. The ovary has a hilus. Also called a *hilum.*

Homologous   Two organs that have similar structure, position, and origin.

Homologous chromosomes   Two chromosomes that belong to a pair. Each pair has a paternal chromosome (from the father) and a maternal chromosome (from the mother). Also called *homologues.*

Homologues   *See* Homologous chromosomes.

hPL   *See* Human chorionic somatomammotropin.

Human chorionic gonadotropin (hCG)   A hormone secreted by the chorion of the developing placenta. It maintains the corpus luteum during the first three months of pregnancy. From the 4th through the 9th month, the placenta takes over the function of the the corpus luteum (secretion of estrogen and progesterone).

Human chorionic somatomammotropin (hCS)   A hormone secreted by the chorion of the developing placenta. It maintains the corpus luteum. It prepares breast tissue for lactation, causes growth, maintains high plasma glucose levels, and mobilizes fat. Also called *human placental lactogen (hPL).*

Human placental lactogen (hPL)   *See* Human chorionic somatomammotropin.

Hyaluronic acid   An extracellular material that binds cells together, lubricates joints, and maintains the shape of eyeballs.

Hyaluronidase   An enzyme that breaks down hyaluronic acid. It is secreted from the acrosomes of spermatozoa; it digests the material covering the ovum (the zona pellucida).

Hymen   A thin fold of mucous membrane that forms a border around the vaginal orifice (opening), partially closing it. It is usually torn and destroyed by the first sexual intercourse.

ICSH   *See* Luteinizing hormone.

Identical twins   *See* Monozygotic twins.

Implantation   Attachment of the blastocyst to the lining of the uterus (endometrium) about one week after fertilization.

Induced abortion   A birth control method. The surgical or drug-induced removal of the embryo.

Inferior vena cava   Large vein that collects blood from the parts of the body inferior to the heart. It empties into the right atrium of the heart.

Infundibulum   Two definitions. In the female reproductive system, the infundibulum is the funnel-shaped distal end of the uterine (Fallopian) tube. It is also the stalklike structure that attaches the pituitary gland to the hypothalamus.

Inguinal   Pertaining to the groin.

Inguinal canal   An oblique passageway in the anterior abdominal wall just superior and parallel to the medial half of the inguinal ligament. In males, the spermatic cord and ilioinguinal nerve pass through the inguinal canal; in females, the round ligament of the uterus and the ilioinguinal nerve pass through the inguinal canal.

Inhibin   A hormone secreted by the corpus luteum. It inhibits the secetion of gonadotropin-releasing hormone (GnRH) and follicle-stimulating hormone (FSH) from the hypothalamus and anterior pituitary gland, respectively.

Inner cell mass   A mass of cells inside the blastocyst that differentiates into the primary germ layers (ectoderm, mesoderm, and endoderm). Also called the *embryoblast.*

Internal iliac arteries   Branches of the abdominal aorta that carry blood toward the legs. In the female, branches of these arteries supply the uterus. During fetal development, blood passes from the fetus to the placenta via umbilical arteries, which branch from the internal iliac arteries.

Internal os   The narrow opening between the uterine cavity and the cervical canal.

Interstitial cell of Leydig   *See* Interstitial endocrinocyte.

Interstitial cell stimulating hormone (ICSH)   *See* Luteinizing hormone.

Interstitial endocrinocyte   A cell located in the connective tissue between seminiferous tubules; it secretes the male hormone testosterone. Also called *interstitial cell of Leydig.*

Intervillous space   The region of the decidua basalis located between chorionic villi in the placenta. It contains contains sinuses (spaces) filled with maternal blood.

Intrauterine device (IUD)   A device used for birth control. A small object made of plastic, copper, or stainless steel is inserted into the cavity of the uterus; it blocks implantation.

Isthmus   A narrow strip of tissue or narrow passageway connecting two larger parts. The isthmus of the uterine tube is the constricted portion that attaches to the uterus; the isthmus of the uterus is the constricted portion that marks the junction between the body and the cervix of the uterus.

IUD   *See* Intrauterine device.

Labia majora   (singular: labium majus)   Two longitudinal folds of skin extending inferiorly and posteriorly from the mons pubis of the female.

Labia minora   (singular: labium minus)   Two small folds of mucous membrane lying medial to the labia majora of the female.

Labium   (plural: labia)   A lip or liplike structure.

Labor   The process of giving birth. Also called *childbirth*, *parturition*, *delivery*, *confinement*, and *travail*.

Lactation   The secretion and ejection of milk by the mammary glands.

Lactiferous duct   A tube that carries milk from a lactiferous sinus to the exterior of a nipple.

Lactiferous sinus   An expanded portion of a mammary duct near the nipple.

Lactogenic hormone   *See* Prolactin.

Lateral cervical ligaments   *See* Cardinal ligaments.

Lesser vestibular glands   Paired mucus-secreting glands that have ducts that open on either side of the urethral orifice into the vestibule of the vulva (in the female).

LH   *See* Luteinizing hormone.

Ligament   Connective tissue that attaches bone to bone.

Littré glands   *See* Urethral glands.

Lobe   A compartment of a mammary gland. Each mammary gland consists of 15 to 20 lobes separated by adipose (fat) tissue.

Lobule   In the mammary glands, a lobule is a mass of connective tissue in which milk-secreting glands are embedded. Subdivisions of a lobe.

Luteal phase   A phase of the ovarian cycle. Days 14 to 28 of the ovarian cycle. The period of time when the corpus luteum is functioning.

Luteinizing hormone (LH)   A hormone (gonadotropin) secreted by the anterior pituitary gland. In females, an LH surge on the fourteenth day stimulates ovulation; after ovulation, low levels of LH stimulate the corpus luteum to secrete estrogen and progesterone. In males, LH stimulates the interstitial endocrinocytes in the testes to secrete the male hormone testosterone. In males, it is also called *interstitial cell stimulating hormone (ICSH)*.

Mammary   Pertaining to a female breast.

Mammary duct   A duct that carries milk from a secondary tubule to a lactiferous sinus.

Mammary glands   Modified sudoriferous (sweat) glands that are specialized to produce milk.

Mammography   Examination of the breasts by x–rays.

Mature follicle   *See* Vesicular ovarian follicle.

Mature ovum   *See* Ovum.

Meiosis   A type of cell division that produces gametes (sperm and ova). It has two phases, meiosis I and meiosis II.

Membranous urethra   The middle portion of the male urethra. It passes through the urogenital diaphragm (a structure that strengthens the pelvic floor and consists of the deep transverse perineus muscle, the urethral sphincter, and a fibrous membrane).

Menarche   The onset, at puberty, of menstrual cycling.

Menopause   The cessation of menstrual cycling.

Menses   *See* Menstrual phase.

Menstrual cycle   A series of changes in the endometrium of a nonpregnant female that prepares the lining of the uterus to receive a fertilized ovum. It lasts about 28 days.

Menstrual period   *See* Menstrual phase.

Menstrual phase   The first five days of the menstrual cycle. Also called *menstruation* or *menses* or *menstrual period*.

Menstruation   *See* Menstrual phase.

Mesoderm   One of the three primary germ layers in the embryo. It gives rise to connective tissues, bones, muscles, blood, and blood vessels.

Mesovarium   A short fold of peritoneum that attaches an ovary to the broad ligament of the uterus.

Mitosis   A type of cell division. Chromosomes in the nucleus duplicate and then separate, forming two daughter cells that are genetically identical.

Mittelschmerz   An abdominal pain that indicates ovulation (the release of a secondary oocyte from the ovary).

Monozygotic twins   Twins that develop from a single fertilized ovum that splits at an early stage in development. Also called *identical twins*.

Mons pubis   The rounded elevation located anterior to the pubic symphysis in the female; consists of a pad of fatty connective tissue.

Morphology   The study of the form or shape of a structure.

Morula   The solid mass of cells (blastomeres) that form as the result of cleavage about four days after fertilization.

Motility   Movement. The activity of sperm.

Mucosa   *See* Mucous membrane.

Mucous membrane   A membrane that lines a body cavity that opens to the exterior. Also called the *mucosa*.

Mucus   The thick fluid secretion of mucous glands and mucous membranes.

Muscularis   A muscle layer of an organ.

Myoepithelial cells   Contractile cells that surround the walls of alveoli in mammary glands. When stimulated by the hormone oxytocin (OT), they contract; this compresses the alveoli and ejects milk into the ducts.

Myoid   Resembling a muscle.

Myometrium   The smooth muscle layer of the uterus. Located betweeen the endometrium and the perimetrium.

Navel   *See* Umbilicus.

Neonatal period   Pertaining to the first four weeks following birth.

Nipple   The pigmented, wrinkled projection on the surface of the mammary gland. It is the location of the openings of the lactiferous ducts for milk release.

Norplant   A birth control method. Six capsules containing a chemical similar to progesterone that are surgically implanted under the skin of the arm. The chemical, which is released over five years, inhibits ovulation.

Obstetrics   The branch of medicine that deals with pregnancy, labor, and the period of time immediately following delivery (the neonatal period).

OC   *See* Oral contraceptive.

Oocyte   A developing ovum. A primary oocyte is formed by the differentiation of an oogonium. A secondary oocyte is the result of the meiotic division (meiosis I) of a primary oocyte.

Oogenesis   The formation and development of the ovum.

Oogonia   (singular: oogonium)   Diploid cells in the ovaries that grow and differentiate into primary oocytes during fetal development.

Oral contraceptive (OC)   A birth control method. Pills that contain a high concentration of progesterone and a low concentration of estrogen, causing a negative feedback effect on the hypothalamus and anterior pituitary gland; the resulting low levels of FSH and LH prevent the development of a new follicle. Also called *"the pill."*

Orgasm   The culmination (climax) of sexual stimulation. In the male, it occurs during ejaculation; in the female, it involves the involuntary contraction of the perineal muscles. It is accompanied by a feeling of physiological and psychological release.

Ovarian cycle   A monthly series of events in the ovary associated with the maturation of an ovum.

Ovarian follicle   A general name for any oocyte with its surrounding granulosa (follicular) cells. It includes primordial follicles, primary follicles, secondary follicles, and vesicular ovarian follicles (Graafian or mature follicles).

Ovarian ligament   A rounded cord of connective tissue that attaches the ovary to the uterus.

Ovary   The female gonad. One of a pair of structures that produces ova and sex hormones.

Oviduct   *See* Uterine tube.

Ovulation   The rupture of a vesicular ovarian (Graafian) follicle. A secondary oocyte is propelled into the opening (infundibulum) of the nearby uterine tube.

Ovum   (plural: ova)   The daughter cell that is formed by meiosis II. Penetration of a secondary oocyte (in metaphase of meiosis II) by a sperm triggers the completion of meiosis II. The two daughter cells produced include a second polar body and an ovum. Also called a *mature ovum* or *egg*.

Paraurethral glands   Glands embedded in the wall of the female urethra that secrete mucus. They are homologous to the male prostate gland. Also called *Skene's glands*.

Parturition   *See* Labor.

Pelvic diaphragm   A sheet of skeletal muscle that forms the floor of the pelvis. It helps to support the internal organs (viscera) of the abdominal and pelvic cavities.

Penis   The male organ of copulation and of urinary excretion.

Perimetrium   The outer covering (serosa) of the uterus.

Perineum   The pelvic floor. In the male, the space between the anus and the scrotum; in the female, the space between the anus and the vulva.

Peristalsis   Successive rhythmic contractions along the wall of a hollow muscular structure.

PGs   *See* Prostaglandins.

Placenta   A structure that allows for the exchange of materials between the blood of the mother and the fetus. It consists of the chorionic villi of the embryo and the underlying endometrium of the mother. Also called *afterbirth*.

Placental estrogen   Estrogen secreted by the placenta during pregnancy.

Placental progesterone   Progesterone secreted by the placenta during pregnancy.

Polar body   The smaller cell resulting from the meiotic division of an oocyte. The polar body has no function and disintegrates.

Polyspermy   Fertilization of a secondary oocyte by more than one sperm. Normally, after one sperm penetrates an oocyte, calcium ions released inside the oocyte promote changes that block the entrance of other sperm (polyspermy).

Postovulatory phase   The period of time between ovulation and the onset of the next menstruation. Days 15 – 28. With reference to the ovaries, the postovulatory phase is called the *luteal phase*, because the corpus luteum is functioning; with reference to the uterus, it is called the *secretory phase*, because of the secretory activity of the endometrial glands.

Preovulatory phase   The period of time between menstruation and ovulation. Days 6 – 13. With reference to the uterus, the preovulatory phase is called the *proliferative phase*, because the endometrium is proliferating (growing).

Prepuce   The loose-fitting skin covering the glans of the penis and clitoris. Also called the *foreskin*.

Primary follicle   A primary oocyte surrounded by multiple layers of granulosa (follicular) cells.

Primary germ layers   The three embryonic tissues from which all tissues and organs of the body will eventually develop. They include the ectoderm, mesoderm, and endoderm.

Primary oocyte   A diploid cell that results from the growth and differentiation of an oogonium. A primary oocyte surrounded by multiple layers of granulosa (follicular) cells is called a primary follicle.

Primary spermatocyte   A diploid cell that results from the growth and differentiation of a spermatogonium.

Primordial follicle   A primary oocyte surrounded by a single layer of granulosa (follicular) cells.

Progesterone   A hormone secreted primarily by the corpus luteum (in females). After implantation, it maintains the endometrium and prepares the breasts to secrete milk.

Prolactin (PRL)   A hormone secreted by the anterior pituitary gland (in females). It initiates and maintains milk secretion by the mammary glands. Also called *lactogenic hormone*.

Proliferation   Rapid and repeated reproduction of new parts. Cell division, resulting in growth.

Proliferative phase   A phase of the uterine cycle. Days 6 – 13, when the endometrium is proliferating (growing). Also called the *preovulatory phase*.

Pronuclei   After a sperm penetrates a secondary oocyte, meiosis II is completed, forming an ovum. The nucleus of the ovum and the sperm are called pronuclei and have the haploid number of chromosomes (23). The pronuclei fuse to form a diploid nucleus called the segmentation nucleus (the cell is then called a zygote).

Prostaglandins (PGs)   Hormones that have a broad range of activities. In males, prostaglandins are present in the fluid secreted by the seminal vesicles.

Prostate gland   A single, doughnut-shaped gland present in the male; it surrounds the superior portion of the urethra (prostatic urethra). It secretes a milky, slightly acidic fluid that contains several enzymes into the urethra.

Prostatic urethra   The portion of the urethra that passes through the prostate gland.

136

Puberty   Attainment of sexual maturity. Three to five years of sexual development, usually between ages 10 and 17.

Pubic symphysis   A cartilaginous joint between the anterior surfaces of the pubic bones (in males and females).

Pudendum   *See* Vulva.

Radial arteries   In the uterus, radial arteries branch from arcuate arteries and penetrate the myometrium.

Random distribution   The random distribution of maternal and paternal chromosomes during meiosis I. It contributes to the genetic variability of the daughter cells.

Rectouterine pouch   A pocket formed by the parietal peritoneum in the female. Located between the rectum and the uterus.

Rectum   The final seven inches of the gastrointestinal tract; from the sigmoid colon to the anus.

Relaxin   A hormone secreted by the placenta and the ovaries. Near the time of delivery, it relaxes the pubic symphysis and dilates the cervix.

Reproduction   Two definitions. The formation of new cells for growth, repair, or replacement. The production of a new individual.

Rete testis   A network of tubes in each testis (of the male); it receives spermatozoa from the straight tubules.

Reticulum   A network.

Retroflexion   A malposition of the uterus in which it is tilted posteriorly.

Rhythm method   A birth control method. The avoidance of sexual intercourse for about seven days (just before and after ovulation).

Root of penis   The attached portion of the penis.

Round ligament   A band of fibrous tissue enclosed between the folds of the broad ligament of the uterus. It emerges just below the uterine (Fallopian) tube, extends laterally along the pelvic wall, penetrates the abdominal wall through the deep inguinal ring, and ends in the labia majora.

Rugae (singular: ruga)   Large folds in the lining of an empty, hollow organ. They are present in the vagina.

Scrotum   A skin-covered pouch that contains the testes and their accessory structures.

Secondary follicle   A secondary oocyte surrounded by numerous granulosa (follicular) cells that have secreted a fluid, forming a fluid-filled cavity called the antrum.

Secondary oocyte   A haploid cell that results when a primary oocyte completes meiosis I. When a primary oocyte divides during meiosis I, the daughter cells include one secondary oocyte and the first polar body.

Secondary spermatocyte   A haploid cell that results when a primary spermatocyte completes meiosis I.

Secondary tubule   In the mammary gland, a secondary tubule carries milk from an alveolus (milk-secreting gland) to a mammary duct.

Secretion   In the mammary glands, secretion refers to the release of milk into the alveoli, which become dilated. It is stimulated by the hormone prolactin (PRL), which is secreted by the anterior pituitary gland.

Secretory phase   A phase of the uterine cycle. Days 15 – 28, when the endometrial glands are actively secreting. It is the same period as the *luteal phase* of the ovarian cycle and the *postovulatory phase* of the reproductive cycle.

Segmentation nucleus   The diploid nucleus of a zygote.

Semen   The fluid discharged by a male during ejaculation. It consists of spermatozoa and secretions of the seminal vesicles, prostate gland, and bulbourethral (Cowper's) glands.

Seminal duct   *See* Ductus deferens.

Seminal plasmin   An antibiotic present in semen.

Seminiferous tubule   A tightly coiled tubule located in the lobule of a testis, where spermatozoa are produced.

Septum (plural: septa)   A wall (partition) dividing two spaces.

Sertoli cell   *See* Sustentacular cell.

Sex chromosomes   The chromosomes that determine the sex of an individual. The 23rd pair of chromosomes. In males, the pair is XY; in females, the pair is XX.

Sexual intercourse   The insertion of the erect penis into the vagina. Also called *coitus* and *copulation*.

Skene's glands   *See* Paraurethral glands.

Sperm   *See* Spermatozoon.

Spermatic cord   The ductus deferens with its associated structures (testicular artery, autonomic nerves, veins, lymphatic vessels, and cremaster muscle).

Spermatid   The haploid cell found in the testes (of the male) that results when a secondary spermatocyte divides by meiosis II. Spermatids differentiate into spermatozoa.

Spermatocyte   A developing spermatozoon found in the testes (of a male). A primary spermatocyte is formed by the differentiation of a spermatogonium. A secondary spermatocyte is the result of the meiotic division (meiosis I) of a primary spermatocyte.

Spermatogenesis   The formation and development of spermatozoa.

Spermatogonia (singular: spermatogonium)   Diploid cells in the testes that grow and differentiate into primary spermatocytes throughout the life of a male.

Spermatozoon (plural: spermatozoa)   A mature sperm cell.

Spermiation   The release of spermatozoa from sustentacular cells into the fluid-filled lumen of a seminiferous tubule.

Spermicide   An agent that kills spermatozoa.

Spermiogenesis   The differentiation of spermatids into spermatozoa. The development of a head, acrosome (enzyme-containing granule), and tail (flagellum)

Sphincter   A ring of smooth muscle surrounding a tube. It functions as a valve; as the muscle contracts, the tube closes.

Spiral arteriole   In the uterus, spiral arterioles branch from radial arteries and supply the stratum functionalis.

Spongy urethra   The portion of the urethra that passes through the corpus spongiosum of the penis.

Sterilization   A method of birth control. In males, a portion of the ductus deferens is surgically removed (vasectomy). In females, a portion of the uterine tube is surgically removed (tubal ligation).

Straight arterioles   In the uterus, straight arterioles branch from radial arteries and supply the stratum basalis.

Straight tubule   A tubule leading from a seminiferous tubule to the rete testis (in the male testis).

Stratum basalis   The permanent portion of the endometrium. Each month it gives rise to a new stratum functionalis, which is shed during menstruation. Also called the *basal layer*.

Stratum functionalis   The layer of the endometrium that is shed during menstruation. Also called the *functional layer*.

Stroma   In the ovary, the stroma is the connective tissue in which the ovarian follicles are embedded.

Superficial inguinal ring A triangular opening in the aponeurosis of the external oblique muscle; it is the end of the inguinal canal.

Suspensory ligaments Two definitions. Suspensory ligaments support the *ovaries*, attaching them to the pelvic wall. The suspensory ligaments that support the *breasts* run between the skin and pectoralis muscle, and are also called *Cooper's ligaments*.

Sustentacular cell Cell found in the wall of a seminiferous tubule that has many functions related to sperm production. Also called a *Sertoli cell*.

Sympto-thermal method A birth control method. The signs of ovulation are used to determine the period of abstinence.

Synapsis The pairing of homologous chromosomes during meiosis I. During synapsis, segments of homologous chromosomes overlap, break, and exchange genes.

Syncytiotrophoblast The portion of the trophoblast that consists of a syncytium (a multinucleate mass of cytoplasm, formed by the fusion of cells). This tissue releases enzymes that dissolve the endometrium during implantation.

Syngamy (*syn* = together) The coming together of gametes. The penetration of a secondary oocyte by a single spermatozoon.

Testicle *See* Testis.

Testis (plural: testes) The male gonad, which produces spermatozoa and the sex hormone testosterone. Also called a *testicle*.

Testosterone The principal androgen (male sex hormone). It is secreted by interstitial endocrinocytes (cells of Leydig), which are located in the testes. It controls the development of male sex organs, secondary sex characteristics, and body growth.

Tetrad A four-chromatid grouping that occurs during meiosis I. Homologous chromosomes (each consisting of two identical chromatids) line up on either side of the equatorial plane.

"The pill" *See* Oral contraceptive.

Travail *See* Labor.

Trophoblast The outer covering of cells of the blastocyst.

Tubal ligation A method of birth control. A surgical procedure that results in the sterilization of females. The uterine tubes are tied and then cut.

Tunica albuginea A dense layer of white fibrous tissue covering a testis or deep to the surface of an ovary.

Tunica vaginalis An outpocketing of the peritoneum that covers each testis. It is superficial to the tunica albuginea.

Umbilical Pertaining to the umbilicus or navel.

Umbilical arteries Two arteries that carry deoxygenated fetal blood through the umbilical cord to the placenta.

Umbilical cord A long, ropelike structure that connects the fetus to the placenta. It consists of one umbilical vein and two umbilical arteries embedded in a connective tissue called Wharton's jelly. It is covered by the amnion.

Umbilical vein A single vein that carries oxygenated blood and nutrients from the placenta to the fetus.

Umbilicus A small scar on the abdomen that marks the former attachment of the umbilical cord to the fetus. Also called the *navel*.

Urethra A small tube leading from the floor of the urinary bladder to the exterior of the body.

Urethral glands Glands in the spongy urethra of the male penis that produce mucus for lubrication during sexual intercourse. Also called *Littré glands*.

Urogenital triangle The region of the pelvic floor bounded by the pubic symphysis and the ischial tuberosities; it contains the external genitalia.

Uterine arteries Branches of the internal iliac arteries that carry blood to the uterus and vagina.

Uterine cavity The space inside the uterus.

Uterine cycle The changes that occur in the uterus during each menstrual cycle.

Uterine tube A duct that transports ova from the ovary to the uterus. Also called *Fallopian tube* or *oviduct*.

Uterine veins Veins that drain blood from the uterus and vagina.

Uterosacral ligaments Peritoneal extensions that connect the uterus to the sacrum.

Uterus The hollow, muscular organ in females that is the site of menstruation, implantation, development of the fetus, and labor. Also called the *womb*.

Vagina A muscular, tubular organ that leads from the uterus to the vestibule. It is located between the urinary bladder and the rectum of the female.

Vaginal orifice External opening of the vagina.

Vaginal pouch A device used for birth control. A polyurethane sheath is placed over the cervix of the uterus. Also called the *female condom*.

Vas deferens *See* Ductus deferens.

Vasectomy A method of birth control. A surgical procedure that results in the sterilization of males. The ductus deferens are tied and then cut.

Vesicle A small bladder or sac containing liquid.

Vesicouterine pouch A pocket formed by the parietal peritoneum in the female. Located between the urinary bladder and the uterus.

Vesicular ovarian follicle A mature follicle. Also called a *Graafian follicle* or *mature follicle*.

Vestibule The cleft (space) between the labia minora in the female. Contains openings of the vagina and the urethra.

Viable Capable of living.

Vulva The external genitalia of the female. Includes the mons pubis, labia majora, labia minora, clitoris, and vestibule. Also called the *pudendum*.

Wharton's jelly Connective tissue in the umbilical cord.

Withdrawal *See* Coitus interruptus.

Womb *See* Uterus.

Yolk sac One of the four embryonic membranes. Nonfunctional in humans.

Zona pellucida A gelatinous glycoprotein layer that surrounds a secondary oocyte. It disintegrates when the blastocyst forms (5th day after fertilization).

Zygote A fertilized ovum with a diploid nucleus.

Bibliography

Curtis, Helena. *Biology,* 3rd ed.
New York : Worth, 1979.

Dorland, William Alexander.   *Dorland's Illustrated Medical Dictionary,* 27th ed.
Philadelphia : W. B. Saunders, 1988.

Ganong, William F.   *Review of Medical Physiology*, 15th ed.
Norwalk, Connecticut : Appleton & Lange, 1991.

Junqueira, L. Carlos, Jose Carneiro, and Robert O. Kelley.   *Basic Histology*, 6th ed.
Norwalk, Connecticut : Appleton & Lange, 1989.

Kapit, Wynn and Lawrence M. Elson.   *The Anatomy Coloring Book.*
New York : HarperCollins, 1977.

Kimball, John W.   *Biology*, 4th ed.
Reading, Massachusetts : Addison-Wesley, 1978.

Melloni, B.J., Ida Dox, and Gilbert Eisner.   *Melloni's Illustrated Medical Dictionary*, 2nd ed.
Baltimore : Williams & Wilkins, 1992.

Moore, Keith L.   *Clinically Oriented Anatomy*, 3rd ed.
Baltimore : Williams & Wilkins, 1992.

Netter, Frank H.   *Atlas of Human Anatomy.*
Summit, N.J. : Ciba–Geigy, 1989.

Tortora, Gerard J. and Sandra Reynolds Grabowski. *Principles of Anatomy and Physiology,* 7th ed.
New York : HarperCollins, 1993.

Vander, Arthur J., James H. Sherman, and Dorothy S. Luciano.   *Human Physiology,* 5th ed.
New York : McGraw-Hill, 1990.